STEVE ADCOCK'S
Partner Workout

STEVE ADCOCK'S
Partner Workout

by Steven Adcock

Photographs by John Bean

M. Evans and Company, Inc.
New York

Library of Congress Cataloging in Publication Data

Adcock, Steven.
  Steve Adcock's partner workout.

  1. Exercise.   2. Physical Fitness.   I. Title.
II. Title: Partner workout.
GV481.A33   1984   613.7   84-13687

ISBN 0-87131-447-9

Copyright © 1984 by Steven Adcock

M. Evans and Company, Inc.
216 East 49 Street
New York, New York 10017

Design by James L. McGuire

Manufactured in the United States of America

9 8 7 6 5 4 3 2 1

This book is dedicated to my daughter, Natane.

Acknowledgments

I would like to thank Mel Roman for giving me the encouragement to write this book, Jack Silverman for his continued support and guidance, and Linda Izzo for being an equal partner.

Contents

	Introduction	11
1	The Adcock System	13
2	Mechanics: Free Weights, Machines, and the Partner Technique	17
3	Breathing and Form, Warm-up, and Freebody Exercises	25
4	Basic Program	48
5	Aerobic Program: Peripheral Heart Action Circuit Training	70
6	Flexibility Program: Proprioceptive Neuromuscular Facilitation	96
7	Advanced Program: Negative Emphasis Training	114
8	Special Training	136
9	Training and Overtraining	187
	Appendix: Muscle Identification	189

Introduction

This book contains an alternative approach, which I began to develop over ten years ago in order to help professional dancers develop upper body strength. Subsequent work with people of every size, shape, and level of fitness has given me the opportunity to create a biomechanical system of movements that can duplicate any resistance exercise that can be done on a machine or with free weights.

There is nothing wrong with working out in a gym with Nautilus equipment, jogging, or lifting weights, but my integrated system of exercise does it all and much more. With my system, your gym is always handy because it's in your own home, hotel room, or vacation house. You can work out wherever you are without battling weather, traffic, or crowds.

With my Partner Workout System, you have a coach at every workout. You don't have to be a professional athlete or spend hundreds of dollars on private instructors and health club memberships to have the support and inspiration that a personal trainer can provide. You and your partner will become each other's coach. Your partner can be a friend, mate, or child—anyone with whom you feel comfortable. Someone you trust. Someone who is reliable, considerate, and as eager to work as you are. Mutual responsibility makes partnering work. You will think twice about missing a workout when someone else's interests are concerned.

My Partner Workout System will transform a solitary pursuit into a social activity. It is "play" in the best sense of the word. You will find that competition, in its limited sense of "beat your opponent," will not succeed in the Partner Workout. Mutual cooperation is necessary to perform the exercises. You will experience the pleasure of touching and being touched. My program will add a sensuous edge that cold machines and barbells cannot. You will become sensitive to each other's body.

The beauty of my system is that it is infinitely variable. You will discover at least two and often more ways to keep yourself and your partner excited about strengthening parts of your body. Your workouts will never become humdrum because you can apply varying resistance, changing "weights," repetitions, and increasing or decreasing speed to each exercise.

As you get stronger, I'll show you how to make the workouts progressively tougher. You'll also learn how to be creative (and thus never bored) through Negative-only routines, Proprioceptive Neuromuscular Facilitation—superstretching—and Circuit Training. You'll appreciate how you can get the same benefits and skill development by using your partner's body as resistance, with the added safety factor that the intelligent "weight" will let up if you feel a cramp or strain coming on.

It's my belief that with a partner you can build the body you'll need for the 80's and 90's. We need a strong, flexible body to meet the challenges of an everchanging world, workplace, and living conditions. We need to communicate better mentally and physically with partners to meet those challenges. My Partner Workout System offers fitness programs to handle our everchanging lives to make us strong and flexible in mind and body.

1 The Adcock System

The Adcock System is an alternative system of exercise that will enable you and your partner to achieve the Four Conditioning Components that are essential to complete balanced fitness: aerobic capacity, strength, flexibility, and skill. With this system, you can develop your own specific goals and work toward achieving a body that is lean, compact, agile, and alert.

The exercises in the Adcock System are designed to help you become more energetic, look and feel better, and move more gracefully. In order to attain more energy, graceful movement, and that feeling of well-being, you must learn to move efficiently. The human body is designed to move. It functions better when it moves, like the engine of a finely tuned race car.

Efficient movement is the result of the interdependence and balance of the mechanics and physiology of the neuromuscular/skeletal system. Your central nervous system gives the command to send the impulse to the muscles. The muscles respond by moving your skeletal structure. All three systems—nervous, muscular, and skeletal—must work in harmony for the greatest efficiency and vitality.

As we all now know, muscles require oxygen to work. In fact, the body's supply of oxygen can be exhausted in only 20 seconds of strenuous activity. When your body's supply of oxygen is depleted, lactic acid accumulates in your blood, and you experience muscle soreness, sometimes becoming quite severe. If your muscles aren't oxygenated immediately, the lactic acid will actually shut down your muscles. They simply won't function.

The point of exercising aerobically, as you have probably heard many times, is to strengthen your heart and make it a more efficient pump—to develop cardiovascular/respiratory fitness. The average adult breathes about 10 to 14 times a minute, exchanging approximately 5 to 7 liters of air. When the body is highly stressed, its pulmonary capacity can increase up to 30 times. However, even at the greatest rate of respiration, oxygen does not necessarily get to the cells to nourish them. The tissues and cells must rely upon the circulatory system, not the lungs, to be oxygenated, and the efficiency of the circulatory system depends not only on the health of its blood vessels but also on the strength of its generator, the heart.

A strong heart pumps more blood with each beat, and therefore has to beat fewer times per minute. Like any other muscle, it is strengthened—made thicker and tougher—by overloading it. Aerobic training builds stronger chest wall muscles and increases the size and number of blood vessels that supply all tissues with oxygen for more energy.

ADCOCK ALTERNATIVE I

Aerobic training is usually achieved by activities such as running, swimming, and cycling, but there is another way. The Adcock Alternative I is called Peripheral Heart Action Circuit Training (Chapter 5).

There are three types of muscular strength—endurance, force, and power, and the intensity of each depends upon the muscle's ability to contract. Muscles should be able to contract long, hard, and fast, and this is achieved by overloading the muscle through progressive resistance training. The amount of overload needed to build the three types of muscular strength is achieved by manipulation of the reps (repetitions of a given exercise) and sets (groups of reps performed without resting).

ADCOCK ALTERNATIVE II

Muscles that contract for a long period of time are said to have *endurance*. Endurance is measured by the length of time or number of repetitions that a muscular contraction can be performed. Downhill skiing, in which the thigh muscles are used to keep the knees bent for a long period of time, is an example of an activity that requires muscle duration. Cross-country skiing, in which the arms and legs continually stroke back and forth, is an example of muscle repetition. Training for endurance should consist of light loads with high reps or, better still, by the Continuous Tension and Peak Contraction methods used in my Basic Program (Chapter 4).

ADCOCK ALTERNATIVE III

A muscle that contracts hard is said to have *force*. Force is the type of strength that results from one maximal, voluntary contraction. The Olympic gymnast who holds the "iron cross" on the Roman rings utilizes this type of strength. Training for force should be with heavy loads and low reps. See my Negative Emphasis Training Program (Chapter 7) for an alternative method.

Muscles that contract fast are said to have *power*. Power is a measure of the amount of work that can be accomplished per unit of time, and it is a combination of strength and speed. The explosive hurl of the javelin thrower is an example of this type of strength. Recent research has shown that training with heavy loads at fast speeds will achieve power. See my Special Training (Chapter 8) for developing this type of strength.

Muscle Strength

Among the physiological benefits of muscular strength are (1) increased thickness and density of bones, especially important to women, who in later years are prone to the dangers of osteoporosis, a thinning of bone mass that can lead to fractures and immobility and (2) increased amounts of connective tissue within the muscle, which slows down the aging process.

Strong muscles, as long as they are exercised through a complete range of motion with proper form and perform flexibility exercises, are more neuromuscularly coordinated. In the next section of this chapter, I will explain how a flexible muscle actually contracts harder. With this underlying level of muscular fitness, every basic motor skill, including agility, coordination, and balance, is automatically improved.

There is little doubt, even in established medical circles, that the body affects the mind and the mind affects the body. A strong body creates a strong mind and a sense of control and perseverance in life. Countless students have told me how my strength-training classes have enabled them to accomplish goals they never thought possible.

Muscle Flexibility

Flexibility is achieved through stretching and should be accomplished by the relaxed, passive pulling out of each muscle to its maximum resting length. Stretching is essential to warm you up and cool you down. When done before and after any vigorous muscular activity, it avoids pulls and cramps and diminishes muscle soreness. Muscle fiber can be stretched to 1.6 times its original length before it tears. When tight muscles are exercised, increased force is transmitted to the tendons. Repeated stress on the tendons can be the underlying cause of tendonitis, a condition frequently seen in runners who fail to stretch sufficiently before and after running.

ADCOCK ALTERNATIVE IV

Stretching heals your body and restores your body's energy by stimulating blood circulation, which removes wastes and other toxins from the cells and replaces them with nutrients to restore the muscle for future work. When you stretch, you are not only stretching muscle tissue, but you are also stretching fascia, tendons, ligaments, nerves, and blood vessels—and some of these tissues are more elastic than others. Working with a partner, performing the exercises in my special Flexibility Program (Chapter 6), you will learn to become sensitive to your muscle response, to avoid overstretching and the torn tissues that can result.

Stretching improves muscular development and strength by lengthening the muscle's range of motion. A flexible muscle has a greater strength of contraction. Stretching a muscle before contracting it gives the muscle a certain amount of elastic, or potential, energy, which gives the following contraction more intensity. And with more intensity, you have a potential for a greater workout.

Muscle Skill

Developing a skill is a motor learning process. It involves the imprinting of codes on our neural circuitry by the repetitive practice of particular movements. When called upon, the master switchboard—our brain—sends these precoded messages via our central nervous system to our muscle tissues, which engage our skeletal system to perform the required task.

The interdependence of the Four Conditioning Components of muscular fitness is clearly demonstrated when they are related to the learning of *skills*. You need muscles that are *flexible* enough to withstand movement in extreme ranges, that are *strong* enough to control and execute the required movements, and are *aerobically* well-fueled to produce enough energy to complete the task. Learning the exercise techniques in the Adcock System will improve total body coordination and balance, and isolated muscle control. The exercises will not improve your tennis serve, per se, but will give you the control and balance necessary to execute movements without wasting muscular effort.

2 Mechanics: Free Weights, Machines, and the Partner Technique

There are literally hundreds of training devices on the market today. We will look at the most publicized and widely used ones and see how they work, and will list their advantages and disadvantages. We will then compare these devices with the advantages of the Adcock System.

FREE WEIGHTS

Free weights consist of barbells, which are long bars 5 to 7 feet in length, and dumbbells, which are short bars from 8 to 14 inches in length. The weights consist of iron plates that slide onto the bars and are attached by collars. A barbell is lifted with both arms and a dumbbell with one arm. Other optional equipment includes racks and benches. The exercises are done by lifting, lowering, pushing, or pulling the weights while the body is in various standing, lying, or squatting positions.

The advantages to free weights are as follows:

1. *Choice of total body or isolated movements.* (a) Total body exercises, such as squats, standing overhead press, and clean and jerk, require maintenance of balance and coordination of major muscle groups, that is, multi-joint involvement such as knee, hip, and shoulder. The result of this kind of exercise is a training of the entire neuromuscular system. (b) Isolated exercises require synergistic energy, that is, fixative muscles that support surrounding areas so that you can isolate a specific muscle. An example of this is the bicep curl, where the shoulder, chest, and back are fixating (supporting) the isolated movement of the bicep. Isolated exercises develop coordination and concentration.

2. *Variety of exercise.* Numerous exercises can be done by changing the hand grip, foot width, and/or body angle. Also, the advantage of using

a dumbbell is that you can train unilaterally, that is, one side of the body, to compensate for any asymmetrical weakness.

3. *Flexibility development.* When free weight exercises are performed properly, that is, through the joint's entire range of motion, flexibility is increased.

4. *Muscular size.* Professional body builders prefer free weights to machines for building muscle mass because greater muscle mass can be achieved.

The disadvantages of free weights are as follows:

1. Handling heavy poundages can be dangerous. Lack of proper gym facilities and spotting techniques can lead to serious injury.

2. The "sticking point" is the weakest point in the range of motion of an exercise, the point where the muscles are at a biomechanical disadvantage. Since the load of free weights remains constant, it is really only at this biomechanically disadvantaged point that muscular contraction is at its fullest. Otherwise, the muscle's level of contraction varies through its "strength curve." In free weight training, there are highly specialized techniques such as forced reps, partial reps, and "cheating methods" to overcome the sticking point problem, but they require hours of practice and professional supervision.

MACHINES

Machines were originally designed in a quest to resolve the free weight "sticking point" problem. All of the controversy surrounding the issue of who makes the best machines revolves around this one muscular goal: maximum muscular contraction.

Universal Machines. According to company public relations, Universal was the first to come up with *the* solution. The Universal system contains a large multi-station machine with up to 16 stations and/or individual machines that work one muscle group at a time. These machines utilize a weight rack with 10-pound increments that are connected by either cables and pulleys or a lifting arm that automatically varies the resistance through the exercise's entire range of motion to coincide with the body's changing leverage. Universal calls this system Dynamic Variable Resistance, but it is also arbitrarily called "accommodating resistance."

Nautilus. Nautilus, now practically the generic name for exercise machines, also uses this accommodating resistance principle. Its mechanical innovation is the Nautilus-shaped cam. According to the company's research, this perfected pulley system *more* closely balances the muscle's movement to achieve an ideal strength curve. The Nautilus setup consists of various self-contained machines, one for each of the specific muscle groups.

Both the Universal and Nautilus machines have a "velocity control" problem. When you lift, pull, or push any weighted object quickly, more effort is required at the beginning of the movement and less as the weight builds momentum against gravity. In resistance training, this lack of pressure on the muscles through their range of motion diminishes contractile effort after the initial thrust. This means that you must exercise on these machines at a predetermined speed. Recent studies show that training with heavy loads at high speeds, if the load on the strength curve is kept constant, will develop complete contraction and a more explosive (quick, powerful) neuromuscular system. With certain standing free weight exercises, such as the clean and jerk, total body power can be developed, but there is a high risk of injury.

Keiser Machines. A recent innovation on the machine scene that successfully deals with the problem of training at high speeds is the isokinetic Keiser Cam II System. The Keiser System, like Nautilus, consists of a circuit of machines to exercise each of the major muscle groups. The machine's mechanical system involves the combination of linkage, bearings, and, sometimes, pulleys that provide accommodating variable resistance and that produce a consistent strength curve over a wide range of exercising speeds. These mechanisms are combined with pneumatic cylinders that contain compressed air. The weight resistance is quantified by pounds per square inch in the cylinders and is controlled by a small, easily accessible pressure valve.

The advantages of machines (Universal, Nautilus, Keiser), in addition to those I've stated so far, are:

1. You can handle heavy loads without the fear of weights falling on you.
2. You can accurately isolate certain muscle groups.
3. You can rehabilitate a certain body part without stressing another.
4. You can work positive and negative "phases." The act of lifting a weight, which involves contracting the muscles, is the positive phase, and the act of lowering the weight, or stretching the muscles while they are contracting, is the negative phase. Both phases are necessary for complete muscle exhaustion.

The same design elements that create the advantages in these machines also create the disadvantages:

1. *Lack of skill development.* Because for the most part you are sitting and strapped into these machines, the work doesn't require much concentration, and no balance or coordination is required or developed.
2. *Lack of variety.* The stationary configuration of the machines and the guided track on which the weights travel, limit the variety and angles with which you can work a muscle.
3. *Design limitation.* The size of the machines and the pivot points that transfer the weights to the handles or footpads are fixed for the average-size person and do not accommodate people of larger or smaller frames, or make them accessible to people with certain other physical differences.

In the end, regardless of the good and bad points I have described about all of this equipment, it all boils down to the fact that the decision to work with machines is based on personal preference, availability, and the specificity of your training goals.

THE PARTNER WORKOUT TECHNIQUE

The biomechanics and physiology of the partnering exercise technique allow you to train with all the advantages of free weights and machines—without any of the disadvantages—plus, much more. Here are some of the things you can achieve with the Partner Workout Technique:

1. *Maximum muscular contraction.* This is achieved by maintaining a smooth, fluid motion throughout the full range of motion of the exercise to compensate for the "sticking point."
2. *Variety.* There are literally an infinite number of exercises that can be done by changing the angle or resistance and by changing your body placement relative to your partner.
3. *Skill.* This is developed by conscious control of angles and resistance.
4. *Velocity control.* The speed can either be maintained or changed through the range of motion, or through the "set," building from slow to fast or vice versa.

5. *Unilateral/bilateral.* One or both limbs can be worked at a time or they can alternate. This is important for developing a weaker side.
6. *Specialized training techniques.* You can work the positive phase only and/or negative phase only.

Before I go on to explain the mechanics of the partner technique, I think that shedding light on how the technique was developed will give you some insight into how valuable these exercises can be for you.

In 1974, I was teaching professional dancers conditioning and rehabilitation at a prominent ballet school in New York City. These dancers all had incredible strength and flexibility in their legs but had no abdominal or upper body development. Ten years ago, the use of weight training was still limited to the realm of body builders. Even if I could have talked these professional dancers into using weights for developing upper body strength, there was no room in the ballet school for such equipment. I started by teaching freebody exercises, such as push-ups and dips. In the search for ways to provide additional resistance, I realized that by pairing people off, and by placing their bodies against one another, I could fixate certain muscle groups and isolate movements to create increased resistance. I soon realized that with some thought, any free weight or machine exercise could be duplicated. Camaraderie among students was an unexpected development. People would show up to class early to "pick their partners." My classes soon became unbelievably popular—they were low cost, there was no hassle of going to a gym, people didn't have to be afraid of being injured on a machine, and they could work with a warm body instead of cold steel. It was a good way to socialize.

In 1980, I founded the Strength Training Institute. For three years, I experimented with various training methods incorporating aerobics, flexibility, and strength training, using this partner technique. The Adcock System presented in these pages represents a total of 14 years of experimenting in the field with over 10,000 students, plus additional research and studies while working on a Ph.D. at Columbia University in Psycho-Social Movement. I have used this system with an incredible variety of people. The blind, young, old, tall, short, theatrical superstars, and professional athletes.

Now let's take a look at how the exercises work. While performing the exercises, we are actually doing work. Work, which is a form of "physical stress," creates the physiological "adaptations" of increased strength, size, flexibility, and improved performance.

According to a law of physics, work equals force times distance

(W = F × D). In resistance training, the specific variables in this formula are: *work*, which is accomplished by multiplying the *force* it takes to move an object, times the *distance* that object has traveled.

An exercise example of this is the military press; the shoulder and tricep muscles are the *force*; the *distance* is the length the resistance travels from the shoulder to a fully extended arm overhead. The amount of *work* accomplished is the number of sets, reps, and so on, and the amount of resistance it takes to achieve muscular fatigue.

The movements we use in resistance exercise are controlled mechanically by a system of human levers and fulcrums. Our muscles act as the force to move the levers (our bones) around a fulcrum (our joints) to lift, lower, push, or pull the source of resistance.

The human body contains three classifications of levers. In the first class of levers, the fulcrum is located between the point at which the force is applied and the weight that is to be moved. An everyday example of this is the seesaw, and an example of this type of lever action in the human body is the extension of the elbow. When a weight is held in the hand, and the forearm is lowered or extended from the elbow, a force (pull) is applied to the ulna (forearm) bone by the contraction of the extensor muscles on the posterior of the upper arm (triceps).

In the second class of levers, the fulcrum is at one end, and the weight to be moved is between the fulcrum and the point of force. The wheelbarrow is a good example of this type of lever, and in the body, a good example is in the bones of the toes: the base of the toes serves as the fulcrum; the toes support the weight, and the force (pull) is caused by the contraction of the posterior muscles of the calf acting upon the heel bone.

The third class of levers are ones in which the weight is at one end, the fulcrum is at the other, and the force is applied between them. The act of lifting a shovel is an example of this type of leverage, and in the body, an example is the flexion of the elbow: the fulcrum is at the elbow joint, the weight is at the wrist or hand, and the force (pull) is made by the contraction of the flexor muscles on the anterior of the arm (bicep). This is the opposite of what occurs in the class one lever example.

The Adcock Technique uses the body's natural system of levers and fulcrums. It creates a source of work (stress) to achieve muscle isolation and resistance in one of three ways:

1. By placing resistance from your partner upon the normal function of the joints.

2. By changing the joint's normal functioning angle
    (a) relative to your body's placement and
    (b) relative to your partner's body position and joint angle.
3. By adding resistance from your partner at this unusual joint angle, in a range through which it would not normally have to move.

It should be noted that these "unusual angles" are well within the joint's normal range of motion. It is just that the joints are not normally used to moving weight through these angles. Isolating the muscles at these angles creates an overload on the muscle, which develops increased strength.

In all three of these mechanical situations, you and your partner can keep the resistance constant as with free weights and/or vary the resistance at appropriate angles for increased mechanical advantage or decreased mechanical disadvantage (sticking point) just as with variable resistance machines such as Nautilus and Universal.

In all of the above situations, you can also change the speed of motion to create accommodating isokinetic resistance. (See Special Training, Chapter 8.)

The resistance that comes from your partner can be (1) equal—same muscle/same angle, (2) unequal—large muscle versus small muscle, two limbs against one, or (3) unusual angle—same muscle versus same muscle—large muscle versus small muscle—two limbs against one. Unlike free weights and machines, the partner technique does not provide precise resistance as measured in pounds. You will, however, still achieve maximum results.

At this point, you may be saying to yourself, "Wow, this all sounds great," but then wondering how you can work with a partner who may be bigger, stronger, or more advanced in training than you are. Over my years of teaching experience, I have found various ways to compensate for these discrepancies in size and strength. You can utilize one or a combination of the following techniques:

1. Pre-exhaustion exercises—for specific muscle used. (Note: see freebody exercises in Chapter 3.)
2. Two hands against one.
3. Use of body weight.

By the way, of all of the muscle groups within the body, the legs are the closest to being equal in cross-sectional width among men and women, so if your partner is of the opposite sex, there shouldn't be any problem in this area. However, if there is, use the following:

1. Pre-exhaustion—freebody exercises (see Chapter 3).
    (a) kneeling front leg lifts (front of thigh)
    (b) lunges (front and back thigh)
    (c) inside leg lifts (inside of thigh)
    (d) straddle squats (inside and outside of thigh).
2. Two hands against one leg unilaterally.
3. Body weight.

3 Breathing and Form, Warm-up, and Freebody Exercises

Before continuing on to the exercise programs, it is important to review the following much-talked-about but little-practiced exercise essentials—breathing, form, and warm-up.

BREATHING

As with many other fine points about fitness training, there is much confusion about proper breathing. There are lots of opinions and myths floating around but few authoritative facts. Some coaches say it doesn't matter how you breathe, just breathe. Others advise you to breathe in through the nose and out through the mouth. And still others insist, breathing through the nose only, to warm the air before it gets to the lungs. As with everything else, there is a right way and a wrong way.

For one thing, breathing through the nose alone requires three times as much energy expenditure as when you breathe through the nose and the mouth. There is a proper way to breathe during resistance exercises. The basic rule is to inhale on the concentric contraction, or when the muscle is shortening, and to exhale on the eccentric contraction, or when the muscle is lengthening. All breathing should be done through the mouth. A good way to remember is to form the letter "O" with your mouth and actually "blow" the air in and out, and don't be afraid to make a little noise. Athletes are often taught to make noise when they exhale to remind themselves not to hold their breath. Making loud noises while exhaling, by the way, as martial arts experts do, also serves to excite additional muscle fiber.

You should *never* hold your breath when doing weight resistance exercises. You can pass out from the phenomenon called the "Valsalva Maneuver." This common, almost subconscious reaction stems from the

25

misconception that when we lift or push a weighted resistance, we should take a deep breath and hold it. We think we are helping stabilize our body, but in fact this breathing maneuver creates a dangerous pressure chamber. This "pressure cooker" effect is caused by bearing down with our abdomen against the air we've just inhaled and then closing off our glottis. The glottis is the opening between the vocal cords through which air enters the larynx. If you have been breathing heavily beforehand, you not only can faint, but you may also raise your blood pressure to dangerous levels, collapse major blood vessels, and even herniate your abdomen.

Concentrate on using your lower abdomen to pump the air. This will take a little practice. A popular misconception in breathing techniques is to expand the rib cage "military" style. This method not only draws insufficient amounts of oxygen into the lungs, but it also distends the middle-back spinal column alignment, interrupting proper nerve flow.

You should inhale by distending your lower abdomen, which will help the diaphragm to contract fully, sucking more air into your lungs. You should exhale by pressing your lower abdomen into your lower back. This isolated abdominal effort will not only exchange greater volumes of air, but it will also strengthen and tone the abdominal wall. A strong abdominal wall helps hold the organs in place and preserves spinal alignment integrity.

The breathing will be slightly different, but not complicated, in each program section. So read the specific instructions at the beginning of each section.

FORM

Proper form during the execution of exercise movements is important for the following three reasons:

1. *Prevention of injury.* Although there are no iron weights, cables, or gears to worry about in the Adcock Partner Workout, you are still dealing with the "weight resistance" of your partner. Movements should always be smooth and concentrated, never jerky or reckless. Concentrated effort during exercise has been shown to improve muscle fiber recruitment.
2. *Proportions and symmetry.* All movements should be complete. No matter what muscle or joint angle you are exercising, complete range of motion is essential. Not only will improper form produce short, bulky, ill-proportioned muscles, but it will also lead to tight, restrictive

connective tissue that will tear easily. Always work the agonist and antagonist evenly (both sides of a muscle joint—bicep/tricep). Overdeveloping one side of a joint will cause a mechanical imbalance, which again will lead to tears and a disproportionate look.

3. *Skill.* The exercises in the Adcock Technique are *isolations*, that is, one muscle or muscle group is exercised at a time. The surrounding muscles remain *fixed* to hold and support the muscle(s) being worked. This muscle isolation and fixation method develops neuromuscular balance and coordination—one of the Four Conditioning Components. In the isolation method, it is particularly important to pay attention to directions such as foot width, arm distance, joint angle, hand grip, and so on. Not following instructions completely can lead to working the wrong muscle. For example, in a chest exercise, bending the elbow the wrong way can produce an exercise that isolates the arm rather than the chest.

WARM-UP

Picture yourself betting on a racehorse, seeing the animal take the lead, and then watching the horse suddenly stop because it pulled a muscle not properly warmed up by its trainers. You'd get pretty heated under the collar, and that's not the kind of warm-up that's very beneficial.

Horseflesh and humanflesh alike need to be warmed up before strenuous activity. The difference is that when you don't warm up and you injure yourself, your money goes to your doctor instead of the betting gate. Besides helping to prevent injury, warm muscles actually contract faster and with more force. Warm ligaments and tendons become more pliable. Heated nerves conduct impulses faster. And warm blood gives up its oxygen more quickly. Efficiency, pure and simple. Horses, humans, and even cars all function better when warmed-up properly.

I have devised 7 partner exercises for the warm-up section. Pick one or combine several. These 7 exercises done continuously for 20 to 30 minutes will also serve as an alternative aerobic workout.

Warm-up means simply that—exercise until you feel warm. You will feel the juices flowing. Do the exercises with light, quick, repetitive motions. Don't strain. Enjoy the warm-up—do it to music. If you feel you want to do a little extra, add some of the freebody exercises in this chapter or pick a few abdominal exercises from Chapter 8, Special Training. Look for specific warm-up instructions at the beginning of each section.

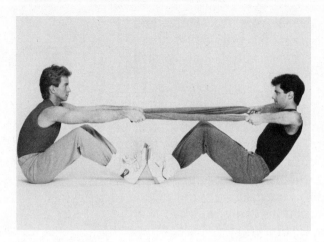 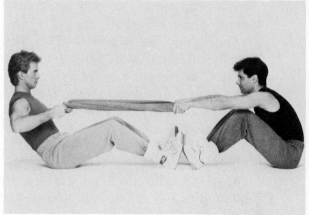

Rowing

Sit facing your partner, knees bent, braced together. Stretch 2 towels between your hands, and, keeping legs stationary, alternate back and forth hip and arm movements with your partner. When leaning back with the hips, bend the arms; when leaning forward, extend the arms. Keep towels parallel to the floor.

Breathing: Rhythmically.

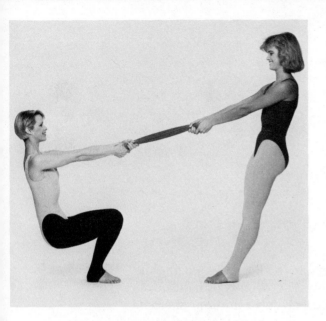 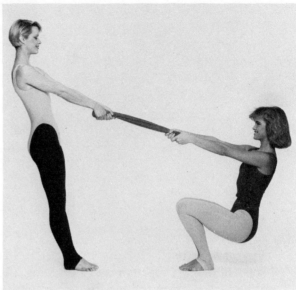

Leaning Seesaw

Stand facing your partner, 3 feet apart. Stretching one towel between your hands, keep arms straight and lean back with shoulders. Alternate up and down knee bends.

Breathing: Rhythmically.

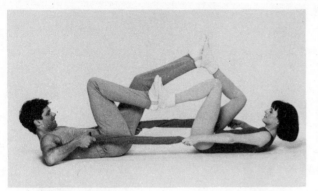 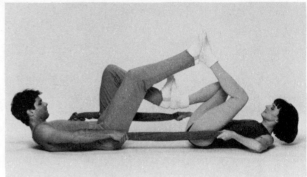

Cycle

Lie on your back facing your partner, 3 feet apart. Begin by placing the soles of the feet together and stretching 2 towels between your hands. While alternating the legs in a rotating back and forth motion, alternate back and forth arm movements parallel to the floor. Maintain resistance between the towels and against the feet.

Breathing: Rhythmically.

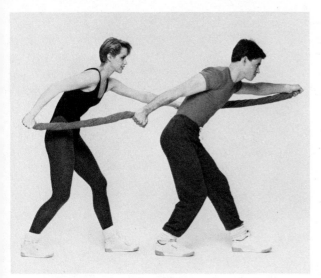 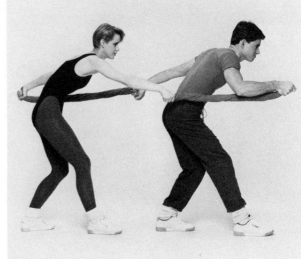

Cross-Country Ski

Stand facing the same direction, 3 feet apart. Stretch 2 towels between hands on either side of body, as shown. Bend from the knees and hips. Maintaining tension between towels for resistance, alternate back and forth arm and leg movements. The leg work is a shuffle-hop step; the arm work is a stiff arm back and forth swing.

Breathing: Rhythmically.

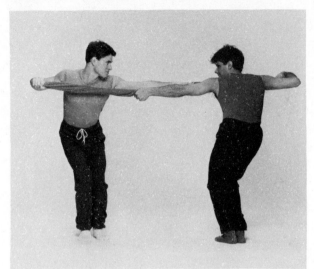 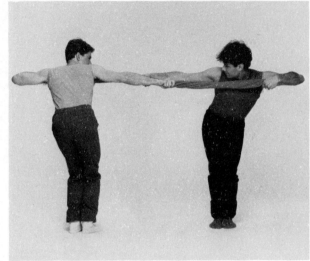

Ski Twist

Stand facing your partner at an angle, about 4 feet apart. Stretch 2 towels between your arms, shoulder height, parallel to the floor. Bend from the knees and hips. Both partners start with left arm extended, right arm bent. Maintaining resistance between the towels, alternate back and forth arm movements, simultaneously coordinated with pivoting the hips, side to side.

Breathing: Rhythmically.

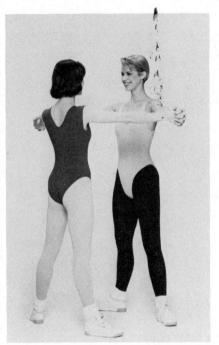 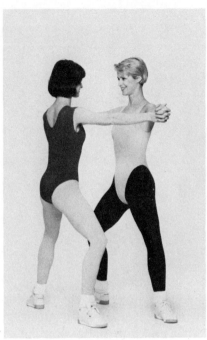 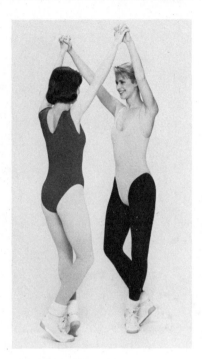

Partner Dance Step

Stand facing your partner, about 1 foot apart. Stretch the arms out parallel
to the floor and interlace the fingers. Begin the step by jumping out to the
side, bending the knees, as shown. Jump back to the center, bringing the
legs together, feet crossed, arms stretched overhead. Alternate jumping to
the side and center.

Breathing: Rhythmically.

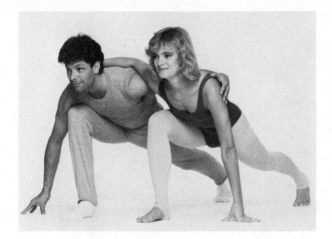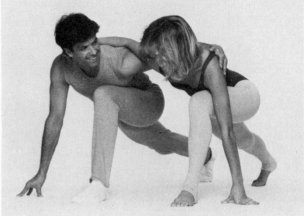

Lunge Thrust

Stand side by side, facing the same direction. Open the legs, front to back, as far as you can. Wrap your inside arm around your partner's shoulders. Begin by bending the right knee and lunging forward, placing your chest on your thigh, as shown. Place outside hand on the floor for balance. Alternate quick back and forth lunging motions with legs kept inside the hand on floor.

Breathing: Rhythmically.

FREEBODY EXERCISES

The 13 exercises are designed to compensate for strength discrepancies in a particular body part that one partner may have. Each exercise caption throughout the book specifies the name of the body part being worked. If, when attempting a particular exercise, you find an unequal strength factor between you and your partner, turn to this section, find the exercise for the body part, pre-exhaust the muscle(s), and immediately go back to the exercise in your program. You may also refer to the Appendix, which has illustrations that identify muscle groups.

Push-ups work the arms, shoulders, chest, back, and stomach muscles. Variations in hand and arm positions isolate and emphasize various muscles. Leg variations redistribute body weight to place more weight emphasis on particular muscle groups.

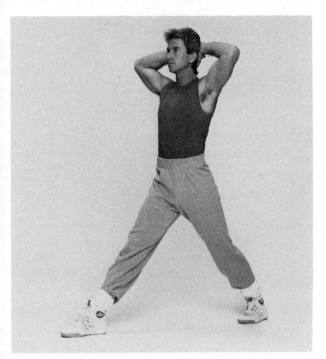 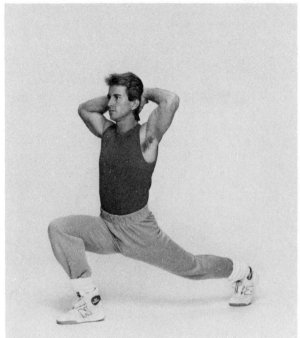

Standing Forward Lunge
(works front and back thighs—quadriceps and hamstrings)

Stand with one foot in front of the other, 30 to 40 inches apart, both feet pointed to the front. Lace the fingers behind the head and open elbows. Lunge forward until the front thigh is parallel to the floor, keeping back leg straight.

Breathing: Inhale as you lunge forward, exhale as you return to starting position.
Reps: 20 times, or until thigh begins to exhaust. Repeat with other leg.

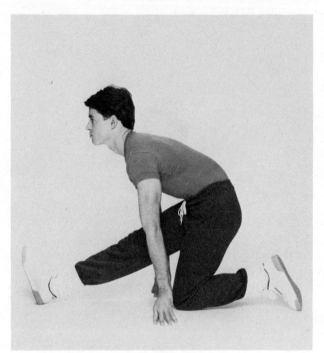
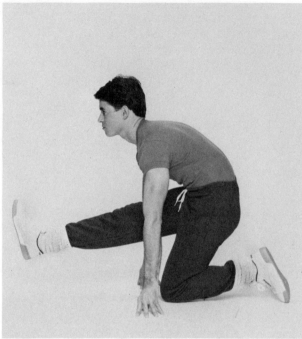

Kneeling Leg Lift
(works quadriceps)

Kneel on one knee and extend the other leg straight in front of you, foot
flexed. Place hands on floor on either side of body to help support body
weight. Without leaning back, lift extended leg.

Breathing: Exhale as you lift the leg, inhale as you lower the leg.
Reps: 10 times should be sufficient to totally exhaust the leg. Repeat with
    other leg.

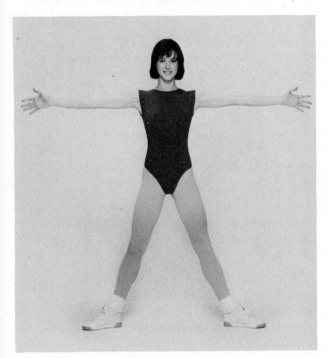
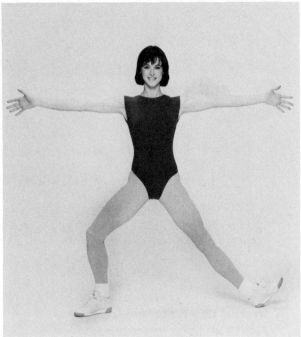

Standing Side Lunge
(works inside and outside thighs)

Stand with feet 24 inches apart, legs turned out. Arms should be
outstretched and parallel to the floor. Lunge to the side, as far as you can,
keeping the heel down. Keep other leg straight and lift toes.

Breathing: Inhale on the lunge, exhale on the return to center.
Reps: Alternate sides 20 times, or until thighs begin to exhaust.

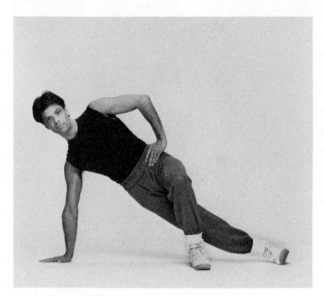
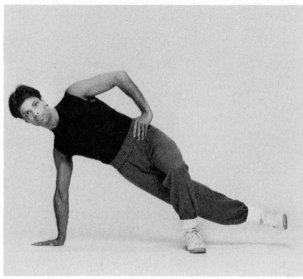

Inside Leg Lift
(works inside thigh muscles)

Lie on your side. Place one hand directly under shoulder, the other hand on hip. Place the foot of the top leg in front of your body, bend the knee, and point the foot to the front, away from the body. Press your body up until arm is fully extended. Do not lean forward. Without lifting the torso or the hips, lift the bottom leg off the floor approximately 6 inches.

Breathing: Exhale as you lift the leg, inhale as you lower the leg.
Reps: 15 times with each leg.

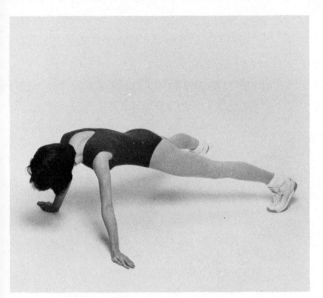
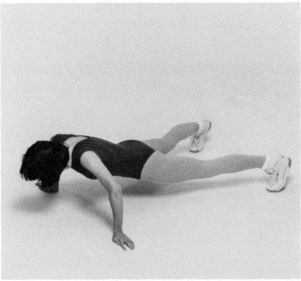

Wide Arm/Wide Leg Push-up
(works chest and middle back)

Place hands, pointed out to the side, 30 inches apart. Open legs approximately the same distance, with the balls of the feet pressed into the floor. Keeping spine and legs straight, lower the body through the arms until the nose touches the floor. Do not lunge head forward to meet the floor first.

Breathing: Inhale as you lower the body, exhale as you press back up.
Reps: 20 times, or until torso begins to tire.

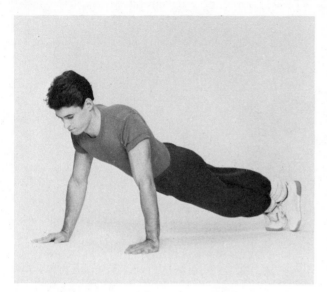
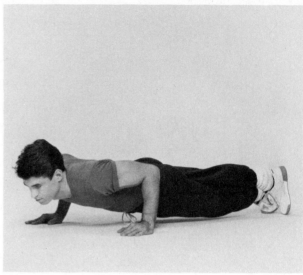

Close Arm/Cross Leg Push-up
(works rear deltoids and triceps)

Place hands on the floor with fingers pointed to the front, approximately 20 inches apart. Cross legs, pressing the ball of one foot into the floor. Do not bend knees. Lower the body and bend the elbows straight back, keeping them close to the body. Keep head, chest, and legs in a straight line. Press body up, extending elbows.

Breathing: Inhale as you lower the body, exhale as you press up.
Reps: 20 times.

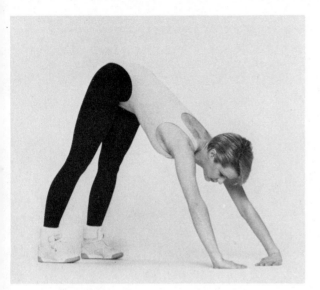 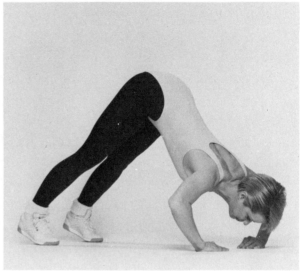

Triangle Push-up
(works trapezius, deltoids, and triceps)

Place feet hip width apart, toes pointed to the front. Place hands, fingers pointed in toward each other, shoulder width apart. Hands should be approximately 30 to 40 inches away from feet. Bend elbows directly to the side until head reaches the floor. Keep legs and back straight.

Breathing: Inhale as you lower the body, exhale as you press up.
Reps: 20 times, or until arms and shoulders begin to tire.

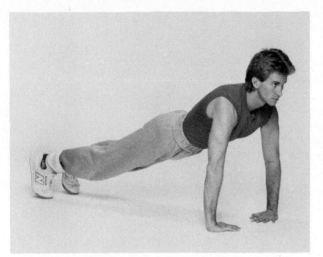 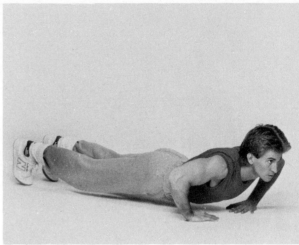

Close Hand Push-up
(works anterior deltoids, chest, and triceps)

Place feet approximately 8 inches apart, balls of the feet pressed into the floor. Place hands on the floor, turned in toward each other under the chest, or approximately 6 inches apart. Lower the body, bending elbows directly to the side, until chest reaches hands. Keep legs, back, and neck in a straight line.

Breathing: Inhale as you lower the body, exhale as you press up.
Reps: 20 times, or until arms or torso begins to tire.

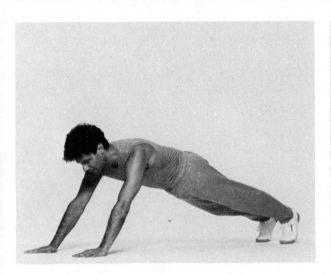 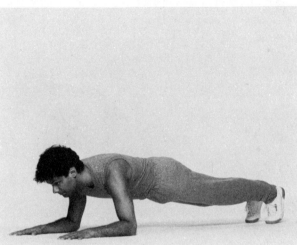

Forearm Push-up
(works triceps, deltoids, and forearms)

Place the hands, shoulder width apart, 12 inches in front of the shoulders. Extend legs straight behind. Keeping the torso and legs in one straight piece, bend your arms, lowering your forearms to the floor. Press up to starting position and repeat.

Breathing: Inhale as you lower, exhale as you press.
Reps: As many times as you can.

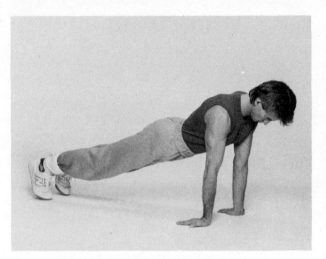
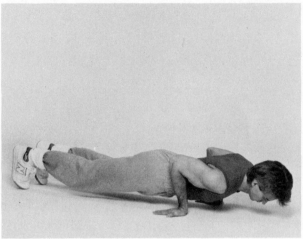

Inverted Hand Push-up
(works biceps, shoulders, and chest)

Place feet approximately 8 inches apart, balls of the feet pressed into the floor. Place hands approximately 20 inches apart, with arms rotated to the back so that the fingers point toward the feet. Lower your body, bending the elbows until the chest reaches the floor. Keep your arms close to your sides so that the elbows point straight back. Straighten the arms, pushing the body back up.

Breathing: Inhale as you lower the body, exhale as you press up.
Reps: 20 times, or until arms or torso begins to tire.

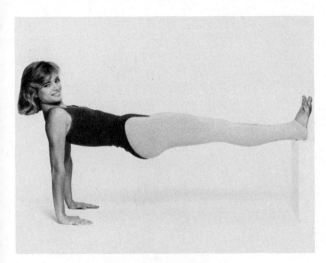
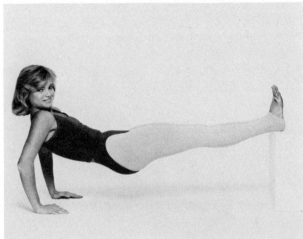

Dips
(works triceps)

Place your feet up on a chair or low table. Position your hands under your shoulders, fingers pointed toward your feet. Begin the exercise by pressing your body up with your arms until your body is parallel to the floor. To exercise the triceps, bend the elbows and lower the hips. Straighten your arms and return to starting position.

Breathing: Inhale as you lower the body, exhale as you press up.
Reps: As many times as you can.

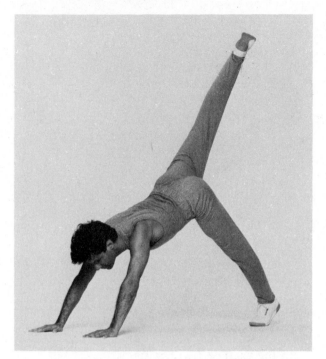 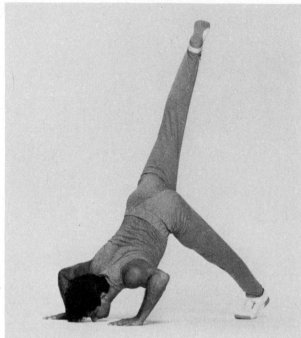

Back Leg Extension Push-up
(works deltoids)

Place the hands in front of your shoulders, fingers pointed forward.
Extend one leg behind and the other leg straight up as high as you can, as
shown. Bend the elbows and lower the head to the floor, keeping the lifted
leg stationary. Press up and repeat.

Breathing: Inhale as you lower the body, exhale as you press up.
Reps: At least 10 times, then alternate legs.

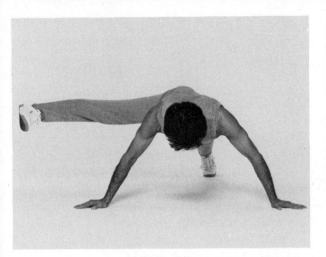
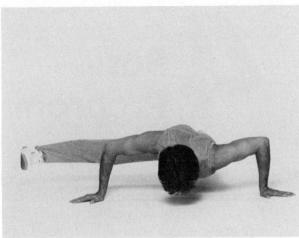

Side Leg Lift Push-up (Advanced)
(works arms, legs, chest, and back)

Extend the arms to the side 3 feet apart, hands pointed out. Extend one leg behind you and the other leg 90° to the side. Press the body and side leg up simultaneously, as shown. Return to about 6 inches from the floor in one solid piece, not the side leg first, and repeat.

Breathing: Inhale as you lower the body, exhale as you press up.
Reps: At least 10 times, then alternate legs.

4 Basic Program

Everyone, regardless of fitness level, should begin with this program. The exercises are designed to be elementary enough for you to learn the required skills of the partner technique, and sophisticated enough for you to achieve a high level of muscular fitness. The exercises work all muscle groups and are ordered in the proper mechanical sequence of largest muscles to smallest muscles.

With this program, the fitness novice will build the foundation of strength in muscle and connective tissue necessary to be able to move on to the more specific fitness goals such as increased muscle size, speed, and agility. The advanced fitness devotee, already possessing a higher degree of strength and skill, can use this program to maintain an existing level of fitness. People of all levels of fitness will find that with the Basic Program they can achieve greater muscular endurance and muscle tone.

Developing fine muscle tone is not just an aesthetic consideration. When muscles are in fine tone, less energy needs to be expended to keep the body erect, and the body is more elastic and less susceptible to injury or to the shock of sudden movement. Dr. Lulu Sweigard, in her book *Human Movement Potential*, compares tonus (the state of tension in a resting muscle) to the idling of an engine. "Good tonus, like the smoothly idling muscle engine, enhances the smooth initiation and performance of muscle work whenever it is needed. The ignition is never turned off."

The 10 lower body and upper body exercises in the Basic Program employ the principles of Continuous Tension and Peak Contraction. Proper form is particularly important in the execution of all movements.

1. *Continuous Tension.* The movements of these exercises should be controlled in a slow, smooth, fluid fashion. Constant tension should be applied throughout the entire range of motion. If you don't maintain the tension throughout the entire range of motion, even when the joint is fully extended, you may slip into a "lock-out" position, in which the pressure of the resistance is being supported by the joint instead of by

the muscle. When this happens, your joints are doing the work that your muscles should be doing, and you don't get the full benefit of the workout.

2. *Peak Contraction.* This concept is closely linked to Continuous Tension. Muscles utilize the greatest number of cells when the joint angle is flexed in a fully contracted position. It is at this juncture that you should apply additional pressure.

The Basic Program, with exercises employing the two movement principles of Continuous Tension and Peak Contraction, will show you how to sculpt a well-defined body. And once you have learned the basic exercise vocabulary of partnering, you will see how it will be possible for you to devise your own exercises for fun and variety.

ORGANIZATION OF THE BASIC PROGRAM

The Basic Program consists of the following:

- 4 additional warm-up exercises:
  2 pre-routine abdomen exercises
  2 flexibility exercises
- 4 lower body exercises
- 6 upper body exercises
- 2 post-routine abdomen exercises (optional)
- 2 post-routine flexibility exercises

Beginners should do the Basic Program 3 days per week (Mon., Wed., Fri.) for 8 to 12 weeks before attempting more advanced exercises. The program should be done for 6 weeks before starting the Aerobic Circuit Training Program (Chapter 5). This will give your connective tissue time to strengthen. If you have a more advanced level of fitness, do the Basic Program for 4 weeks, 3 days per week, before moving on to the more advanced programs.

This program, used 3 times per week by itself, will (1) provide a basic foundation of strength for any rigorous activity, (2) create high-quality muscle tone and endurance, and (3) maintain a high level of existing fitness.

Begin the Basic Program with 5 to 10 minutes of warm-up exercises (see Chapter 3). Then go immediately to the pre-routine abdomen work, and so on. Once you have begun, do not waste time between exercises. Do not leave any more than 2 minutes between exercises. The entire program, including warm-up, should take 45 minutes.

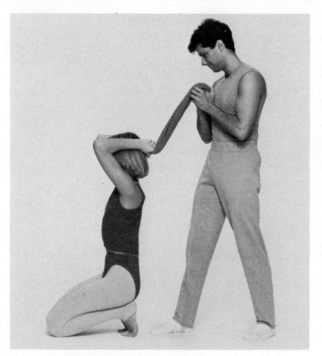
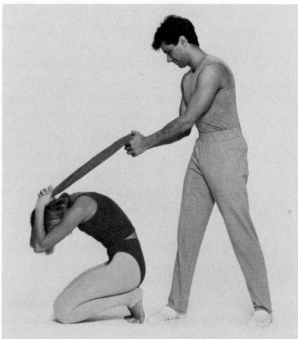

PRE-ROUTINE AB EXERCISE #1

Abdomen Cable "Crunch"
(works upper abdomen)

Kneeling down, sitting on your heels, clasping a towel overhead, as shown, keep elbows bent and stationary. Round the upper back. The assisting partner should stand behind you, holding the other end of the towel at a 45° angle. Maintaining tension on the towel, pull your upper body down toward your knees, exercising the abdomen. Your partner should provide smooth, even resistance with arm and body weight. Release the tension and return to the starting position.

Breathing: Exhale on the way down, inhale on the way up.
Reps: 20 times; then exchange positions with your partner.

Note: This exercise is an abdomen isolation. If, when you bring your torso down, you move your arms from your shoulder or elbow joint, you will be working the wrong muscle.

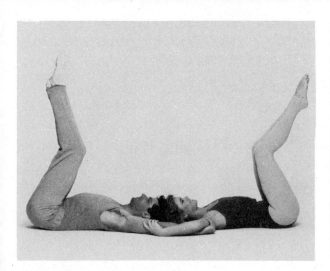 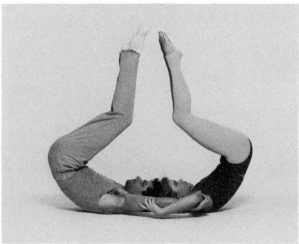

PRE-ROUTINE AB EXERCISE #2

Bent-Knee Shoulder Roll
(works abdomen)

Lie on your backs, head to head, arms extended, clasping your partner's forearms, as shown. Start with legs up, knees bent. Using your partner's arms for balance and support, roll up onto the shoulders, keeping the knees bent, feet pointed, and back rounded. Roll back down to starting position and repeat.

Breathing: Exhale as you roll up, inhale on the way down.
Reps: 20 times.

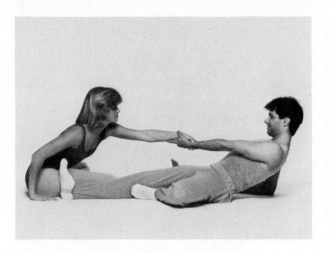 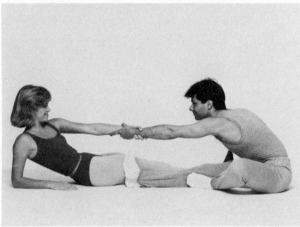

PRE-ROUTINE STRETCH #1

Half-Lotus Pull
(works hamstrings, inner thighs, lower and upper back, and arms)

Sit side by side, extending your right leg, facing your partner. Bend your left knee, placing the sole of the foot on the inside of the right leg. Reach forward and clasp your partner's wrist. Alternate pulling each other back and forth over the extended leg.

Breathing: Exhale as you bend forward, inhale as you go back.

Reps: Each partner stretches 4 times for each leg, holding the extended position for 10 seconds.

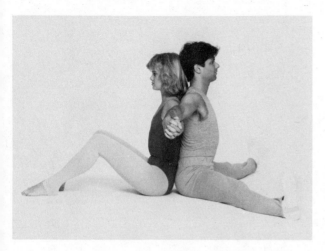 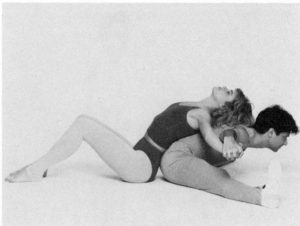

PRE-ROUTINE STRETCH #2

Sitting Abdominal/Inner Thigh Stretch
(works abdominals and inner thighs)

Sit back to back, arms stretched out parallel to the floor, hands clasped.
One partner bends her knees, feet flat on the floor. The other partner
opens his legs in a straddle. The straddle leg partner reaches forward,
bringing his chest to the floor; the other partner lies back, arms and chest
stretched open. Sit back up to starting position and repeat.

Breathing: Exhale on the stretch, inhale on the release.
Reps: 6 times; then exchange places with your partner.

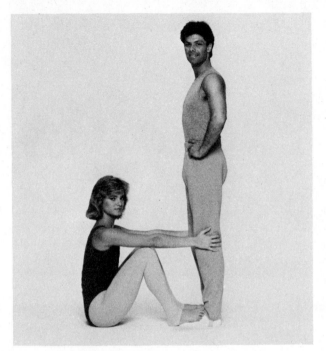 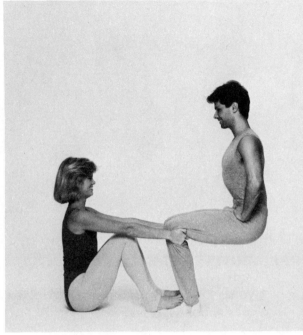

Phantom Chair
(works quadriceps and buttocks)

Stand facing your partner, hands on hips. Your partner assists by sitting
in front of you, knees bent, placing her feet on top of yours, as shown,
and clasping the back of your knee joints. With support from your partner,
lower your hips until your thighs are parallel to the floor. Keep your
calves and back perpendicular to your heels. Do not go any lower than
parallel. Return to standing position and immediately, without "locking"
knees, repeat exercise. Do not rest at standing position. Make exercise
continuous until all repetitions are completed.

Breathing: Inhale on the way down, exhale on the way up.
Reps: 12 times; then change positions with your partner.

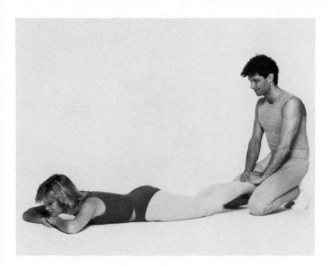 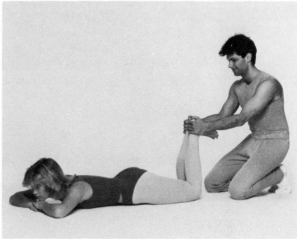

Hamstring Curls
(works hamstrings)

Lie on your stomach, legs together, feet flexed, placing your head on folded hands, as shown. The assisting partner kneels behind you, placing his hands on the back of your ankles. Without arching your back, slowly bend your knees to 90° against your partner's hand resistance. As soon as you reach 90°, your partner pulls your feet back down to starting position, as you resist with your leg muscles. The repetitions should be continuous from beginning to end. Do not pause at extended and bent-knee positions.

Breathing: Exhale on the way up, inhale as you lower.
Reps: 12 times; then change positions with your partner.

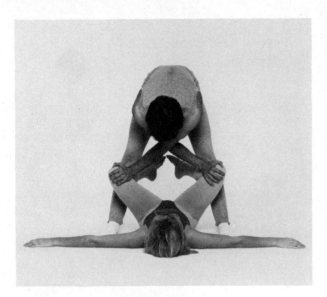
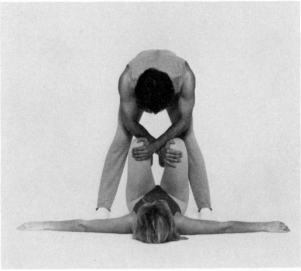

Inner Thigh Adduction
(works inner thighs)

Lie on your back, arms extended to the sides. Bend the legs from hips and knees, and open thighs. The assisting partner stands facing you, bends over, crosses arms and places his hands on the inside of your knees. In a slow four-count motion, bring your knees together against your partner's hand resistance. Release the contraction and return to starting position. Keep the rest of your body stationary.

Breathing: Exhale as you bring the legs together, inhale as you open the legs.
Reps: 12 times; then exchange places with your partner.

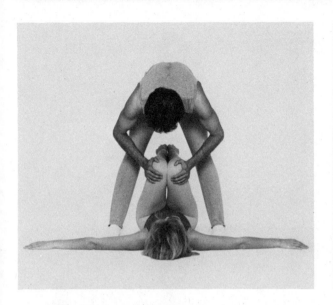

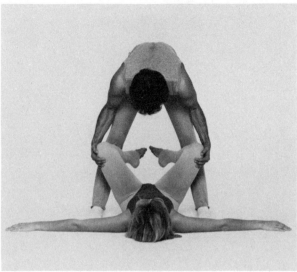

Outer Thigh Abduction
(works outer thigh and buttocks)

Assume the starting position as in the previous adduction exercise, but begin with the legs closed. The assisting partner places his hands on the outside of your knees. The leg motion is exactly opposite from the inner thigh exercise: the work is done by opening the thighs instead of closing them. Release to the center and repeat.

Breathing: Exhale as you open the legs, inhale as you close the legs.
Reps: 12 times; then exchange places with your partner.

Note: The assisting partner receives arm, back, and shoulder work.

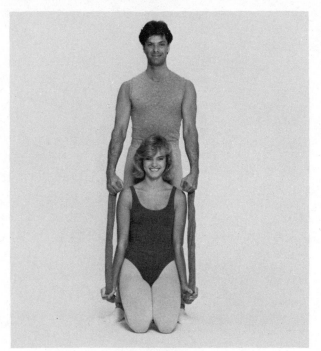 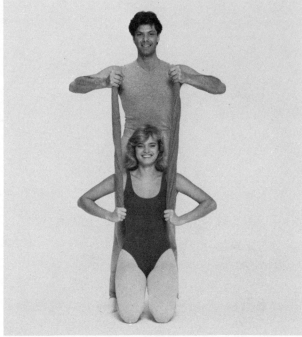

Double Upright Row
(works trapezius and deltoids)

Kneel sitting on your heels, with legs together. Clasp the ends of two towels, extending the arms straight down by your thighs. The assisting partner stands behind you, holding the other ends of the towels with the same arm position. The assisting partner begins by pulling up on the two towels, leading with the elbows, as you, the kneeling partner, provide resistance on the way up—bending the elbows the same way. Then, as soon as you reach the top position, begin to pull down to starting position as the standing partner provides resistance. Movements should be slow and continuous. When you reach the fully extended and bent-arm positions, add a little extra resistance to "peak" the contraction.

Breathing: Exhale on the way up, inhale on the way down.
Reps: 12 times; then exchange places with your partner.

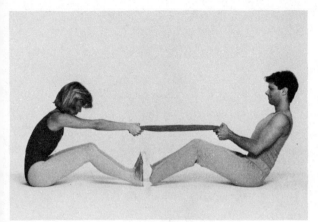 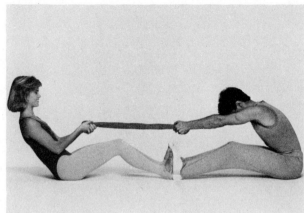

Low Pulley/Bent-over Row
(works latissimus dorsi)

Sit facing your partner, knees bent, feet flexed. Clasping one towel between your hands, alternate back and forth arm and hip movements. As you lean back with your hips, bend your elbows, and as you lean forward, with hips and body, extend your arms. Once you begin the exercise, make the movements nonstop, peaking the contraction when in a fully bent and extended position.

Breathing: Exhale as you lean back, inhale as you lean forward.
Reps: Each partner completes 12 leaning back positions.

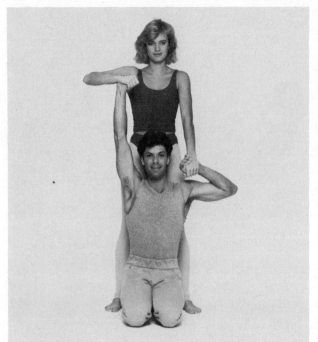 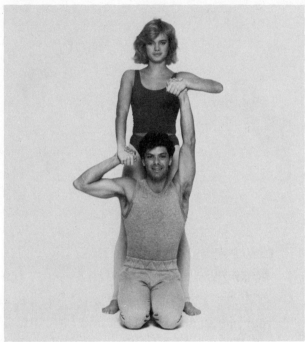

Alternating Military Press
(works deltoids and triceps)

Kneel in front of your partner, clasping hands, extending your right arm up, keeping your left arm down by your shoulder. Simultaneously alternate up and down arm movements, creating resistance against your hands in both directions. Follow the Continuous Tension and Peak Contraction rules discussed in this chapter.

Breathing: Rhythmically.
Reps: 12 extensions per arm.

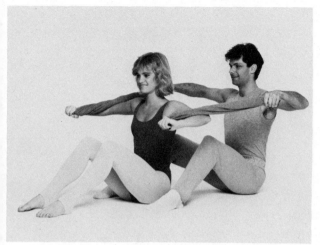 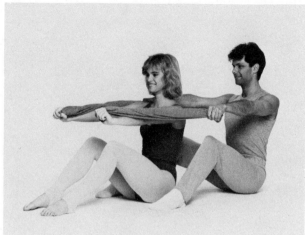

Sitting Chest Press
(works pectorals)

Sit in front of your partner with a straight back, knees bent and slightly open. Clasp the ends of two towels and lift the arms parallel to the floor. Keep the elbows slightly bent. Holding the other ends of the towels, your partner should assume the same back, shoulder, and arm configuration. Resistance is created by your partner, with the towels, when you extend your arms straight forward parallel to the floor. You, then, in turn, create resistance as she pulls back to the starting position.

Breathing: Exhale as the arms go forward, inhale as they go back.
Reps: Arms should be brought forward a total of 12 times; then exchange places with your partner.

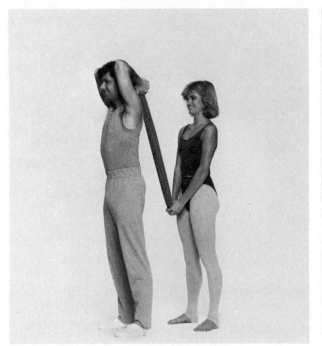 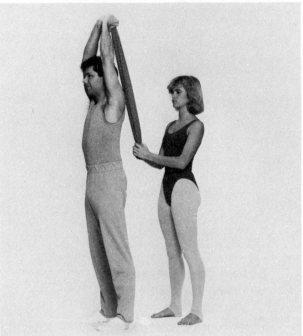

Standing Tricep Extension
(works triceps)

Stand facing the same direction, each clasping the ends of one towel placed between your bodies. The partner in front bends his arms overhead and places his elbows next to his ears, as shown. The partner behind extends her arms straight down in front of her hips. Keeping the shoulder joints stationary, alternate up and down forearm movements from the elbows. Do not use body weight. Stand erect.

Breathing: Rhythmically with movements.
Reps: Each partner extends 12 times; then exchange places with your partner.

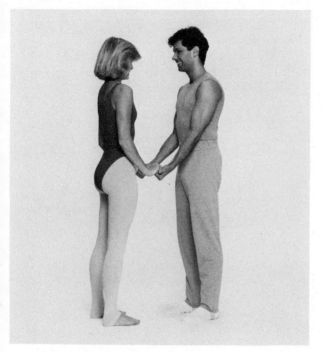 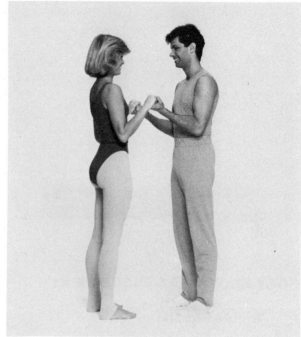

Standing Bicep Curls
(works biceps)

Stand facing your partner, arms extended by your sides, making fists with the hands. Your partner clasps her hands over your fists. Keeping your upper arm stationary, bend your elbows, lifting your fist against your partner's hand resistance. Once you have reached a fully flexed position, resist your partner's downward pressure until you have returned to the starting position. Again, maintain continuous tension.

Breathing: Exhale on the flexion, inhale on the extension.
Reps: 12 times; then change positions with your partner.

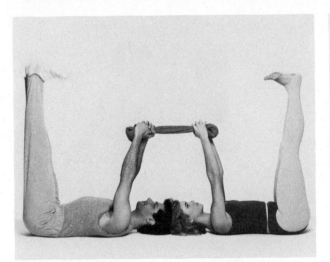 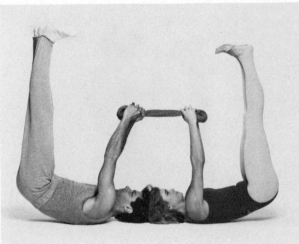

POST-ROUTINE AB EXERCISE #1

Double Hip Lift
(works upper and lower abdomen)

Lie on your back, head to head, arms and legs extended 90° to the floor. Use one towel clasped between your hands for balance and resistance. Keeping your arms stationary and perpendicular to the floor, lift your hips and legs. The difficulty of the exercise comes not only from lifting the hips but also from maintaining a perpendicular leg position. The tendency is to bring the legs back toward the arms.

Breathing: Exhale as you lift the hips up, inhale as you lower the hips.
Reps: 20 times.

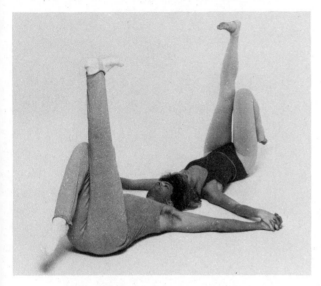 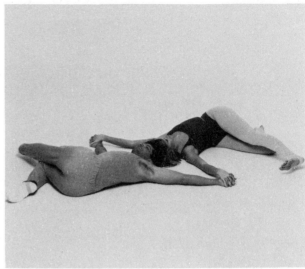

POST-ROUTINE AB EXERCISE #2

One Leg Side Twist
(works abdominals and hips)

Lie on your back, head to head. Extend your arms to the side and clasp your hands, as shown. Bring the legs to a 90° angle to the body. Bend the right knee, keeping the left leg extended straight up. Simultaneously twist the hips and legs to the right side. Return to the center position, change leg positions, as shown, and twist to the other side. Keep shoulders and arms pressed to the floor. Movements should be as coordinated and continuous as possible.

Breathing: Inhale as you lower the leg and twist, exhale as you return to center.
Reps: Alternate twisting sides a total of 6 times.

(Exercise Continues on Next Page)

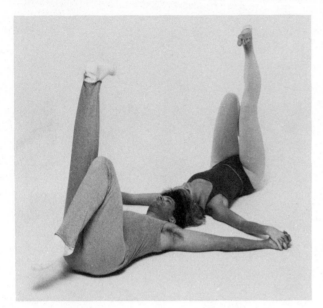 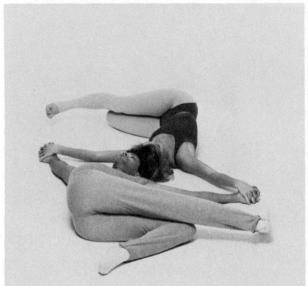

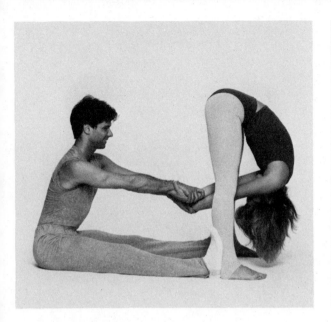 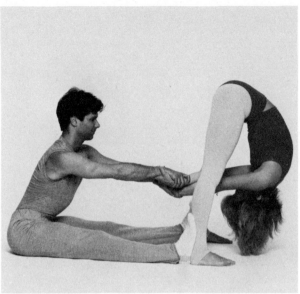

POST-ROUTINE STRETCH #1

Pull-through
(works hamstrings and lower back)

One partner stands, legs open about 3 feet. The other partner sits behind, extending his legs, bracing his feet against the back of your ankles. Bending over from the hip, clasp wrists with your partner. Keeping a tight grip on your partner's wrist, slowly lean forward, stretching your legs and back. Keep chin tucked. Return to starting position and repeat.

Breathing: Exhale as you lean forward, inhale as you return to starting position.

Reps: 6 times, holding each stretch for 10 seconds; then exchange places with your partner.

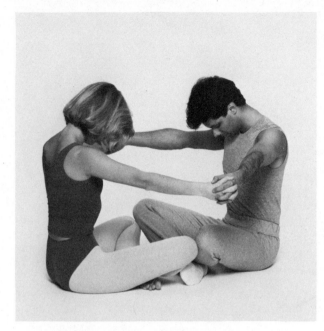 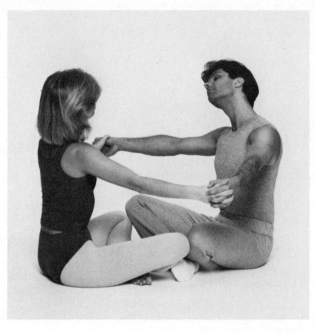

POST-ROUTINE STRETCH #2

Headrolls
(works neck)

Sit facing one another, with legs crossed and arms outstretched parallel to the floor. Lace the fingers together. Both partners start by dropping the head forward and slowly rotating the head to the right, back, left, and then back down to the front. Keep the lower back lifted and the shoulders stabilized.

Breathing: Rhythmically.
Reps: Complete 4 rotations, starting to the right, and then reverse 4 complete rotations, starting to the left.

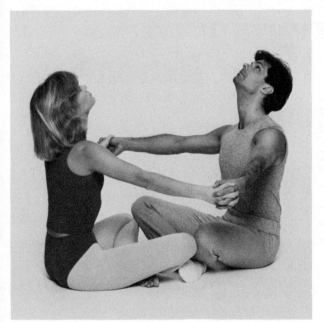
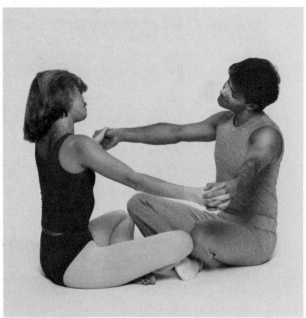

5 Aerobic Program: Peripheral Heart Action Circuit Training

Among the myriad concepts in aerobic training, I've chosen Peripheral Heart Action (PHA) training because it is the most effective way to train utilizing progressive resistance, and it develops cardiovascular/respiratory strength as well as local muscle endurance.

Peripheral Heart Action training was first developed in the mid-1960s by Robert Gajda, a physique star (bodybuilder) with a doctorate in physiology. PHA training was designed to reduce the physique artist's body fat in order to make the musculature more visible. It worked by altering the basic metabolism to burn more calories and utilize digested food more efficiently. Later, it was found that PHA training could be used to develop aerobic capacity and local muscle endurance, and the program I have designed focuses on these two components.

Peripheral Heart Action refers to the skeletal muscles' ability to act as peripheral hearts, contracting to squeeze blood past one-way valves in the vascular system, to aid the heart in circulating the blood. When one part of the body is exercised, blood rushes to that part of the body and pools there, nourishing it and stimulating the growth of capillaries. PHA training is based on the practice of working different and widely spaced body parts (for example, right arm, left leg) in sequence. This forces the heart to work harder to move the blood quickly from one end of the body to the other.

The exercises in this program are performed in a *circuit*, designed to be done in sequence and repeated a specific number of times. If you've been training at a gym, you may have performed circuit training with machines set up in a specific order to work various muscle groups, and moving quickly from one station to another with a minimum of rest in between. The circuit idea is the same here, except that you are moving quickly from exercise to exercise, rather than from machine to machine. The advantage of the partner technique is that you don't have to interrupt your flow and momentum by adjusting machines or changing plates, or waiting for another person to finish at a station. The frustrations of working out in a crowded gym are thus eliminated.

I have designed an aerobic circuit of 15 exercises to be done quickly at 50 percent of resistance, with high reps and very little interval rest in between sets. You'll find that maximum resistance is unnecessary to achieve your goals of aerobic strength and muscle endurance, and that working quickly will develop your speed and your skill. And after this workout, your 62,000 miles of blood vessels will be cleaner, thanks to the increased production of blood buffers—chemicals that cleanse the blood and reduce overall fatigue.

The factor determining the effectiveness of circuit training is *time*. You should work through the exercises at a pace that keeps your heart rate between 60 percent and 85 percent of its maximum. In *Aerobic Weight Training*, Frederick Hatfield, Ph.D., says, "Allowing one's heart rate to fall below the critical value of 60 percent will result in very little (if any) cardiovascular benefit being derived, and working so fast that one's heart rate exceeds roughly 85 percent of his or her maximum heart rate will result in such a diminished capability for sufficient intensity that little strength improvement will be noticed. Further, fatigue will set in before any appreciably aerobic benefit is achieved if one's heart rate is allowed to go too high for any extended period."

ORGANIZATION OF THE AEROBIC CIRCUIT TRAINING PROGRAM

The Peripheral Heart Action Circuit Training Program consists of the following:

- 2 pre-routine flexibility exercises to follow warm-up
- 3 mini-circuits or "Series" of 5 Stations/exercises of nonadjacent body parts:
    - Station 1—Legs
    - Station 2—Back
    - Station 3—Abdomen
    - Station 4—Legs
    - Station 5—Arms
- 2 post-routine stretches

If you are a beginner, complete 6 weeks of the Basic Program (Chapter 4) before moving on to this program. If you are at an advanced level of fitness, complete 4 weeks before attempting this program.

Because little muscle soreness accumulates from this program, it can be done by itself 3 to 5 times per week. You can combine this program with the Basic Program by doing the Basic Program 3 times per week (Mon., Wed., Fri.) and this program on alternating days (Tues., Thurs., optional Sat.).

Begin with a thorough warm-up of 10 solid minutes. During this 10 minutes, elevate your resting pulse rate to your target pulse rate. To find your target pulse, subtract your age from 220, which will give you your maximal heart rate. Your target pulse is then 70 to 85 percent of your maximal heart rate. Once you begin this routine, work nonstop from one station to the next and one series to the next, fast enough to maintain your target heart rate. Check your pulse periodically.

During the execution of the exercise, apply approximately 50 percent of maximum resistance. Don't stop to analyze what 50 percent is; remember, you are working by feel. You will quickly know the difference between maximum effort and less. The individual exercises should be done quickly, while maintaining good form. Don't be reckless. The total program, including warm-up, should take 45 minutes. If you finish sooner, begin with another series. Breathe rhythmically. It is not necessary to take big breaths as in the Basic and Advanced Programs.

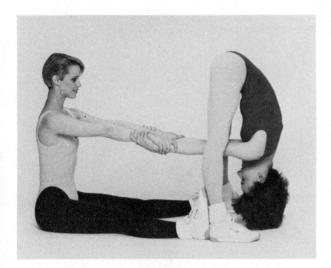
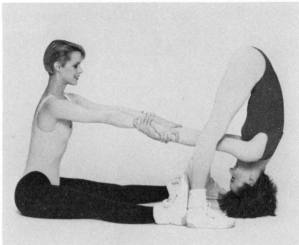

PRE-ROUTINE STRETCH #1

Pull-through
(works hamstrings and lower back)

One partner stands, legs open about 3 feet. The other partner sits behind, extending her legs, bracing her feet against the back of your ankles. Bending over from the hip, clasp wrists with your partner. Keeping a tight grip on your partner's wrists, slowly lean forward, stretching your legs and back. Return to starting position and repeat.

Breathing: Exhale as you lean forward, inhale as you return to starting position.

Reps: 6 times, holding each stretch for 10 seconds; then exchange places with your partner.

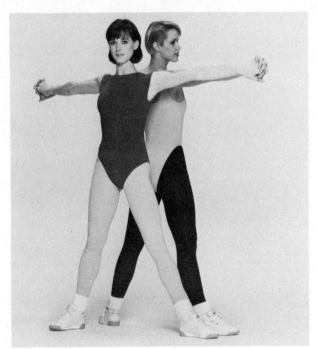 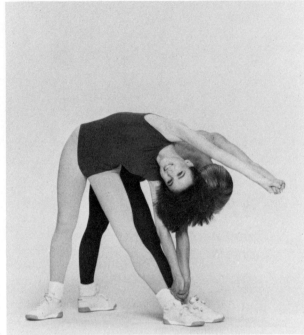

PRE-ROUTINE STRETCH #2

Standing Side Bend
(works inner thighs, waist, shoulders, and arms)

Stand back to back, arms stretched out parallel to the floor, fingers laced together. Open legs 3 feet, front leg and foot turned out, back leg and foot turned parallel. Bend to the side, bringing both arms down, as shown. Return to starting position and repeat.

Breathing: Exhale as you bend over, inhale as you come up.
Reps: Bend 3 times to each side, holding for 10 seconds.

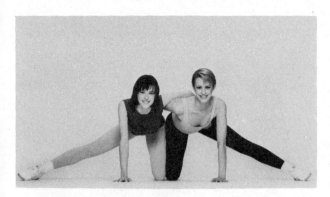
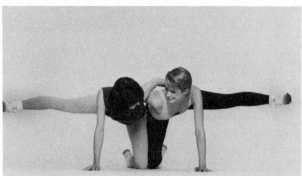

SERIES 1—STATION 1

Kneeling Side Leg Lift
(works the buttocks and outer thighs)

Kneel next to your partner, inside thighs and hips pressing together. Wrap your inside arm around your partner's waist. Extend the outside arm directly beneath the shoulder and the outside leg 90° to your body. Using your partner for balance and resistance, lift the outside leg until it is parallel to the floor. Do not bend the lifting leg or outside elbow. Lower the leg and repeat.

Breathing: Exhale as you lift the leg, inhale as you lower the leg.
Reps: 15 times; then change legs.

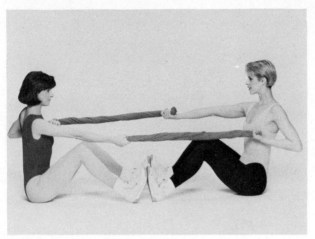 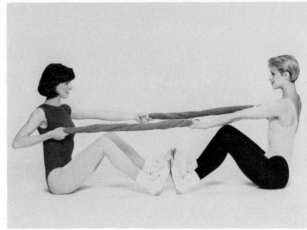

SERIES 1—STATION 2

Sitting Double Arm Pull
(works latissimus dorsi/upper back and biceps)

Sit facing your partner, knees bent, soles of the feet braced against one another. Stretch a towel out in each hand. Keeping a straight back, alternate back and forth arm movements with your partner—bend, extend—bend, extend. Keep arms close to body, with forearms facing down.

Breathing: Rhythmically.
Reps: 12 reps per arm. (One arm bend equals one rep.)

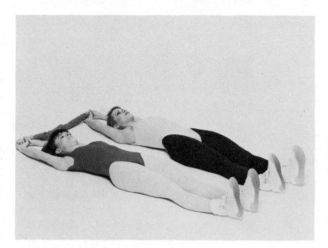 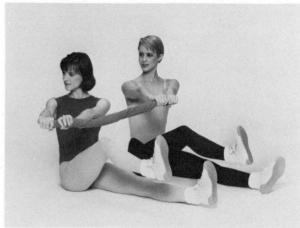

SERIES 1—STATION 3

Sit-up with Arm Twist
(works abdomen and hips)

Begin by lying on your back, one foot away from your partner. Each partner holds opposite ends of a taut towel with both hands above the head. Maintaining the tension between the towels, bring the arms from overhead to the front of the body, simultaneously lifting the torso, twisting to the right, and bending the right knee, as shown. To create added resistance, the partner on the right side pulls the towel to the right along with her twisting torso, and the partner on the left side resists by pulling in the opposite direction. Lie back down to starting position and repeat the same sequence of movements to the left side.

Breathing: Exhale on the way up, inhale on the way down.
Reps: Alternate down, twist right, down, twist left until you have twisted to the right and left 10 times each.

(Exercise Continues on Next Page)

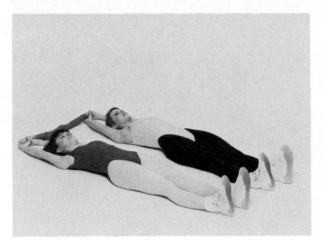 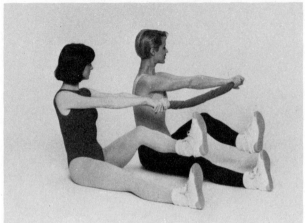

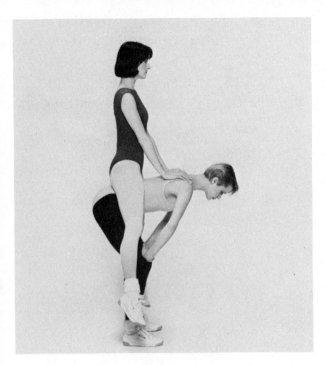
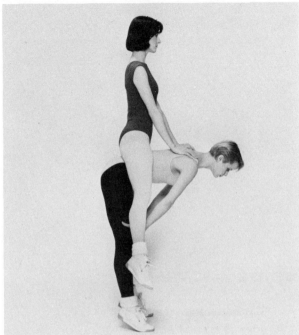

SERIES 1—STATION 4

Bent-over Calf Raises
(works calves, ankles, and feet)

Stand with your legs open hip width. Bend from the waist, making your back parallel to the floor. Bend your knees and place your hands on them. The assisting partner gently climbs onto your back, as shown. The exercise is done by simultaneously rising up onto your toes and straightening your knees. Lower the heels, bend the knees, and repeat.

Breathing: Exhale as you lift up, inhale as you lower down.
Reps: 15 times; then exchange places with your partner.

Note: People with bad backs should do this exercise cautiously.

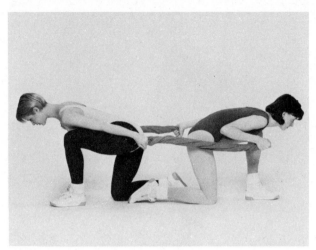 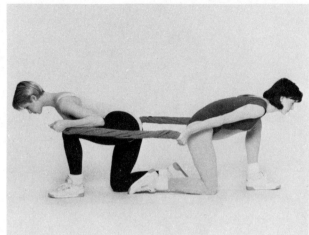

SERIES 1—STATION 5

Kickbacks
(works triceps and biceps)

Facing opposite directions, kneel on the right knee, bend the left knee at a right angle in front of your body. Bend over from your hips, placing the chest inside the left thigh. Stretch two towels between your hands, on either side of your body. Each partner begins with the right arm bent, left arm extended. Keeping the shoulder joint isolated, alternate arm movements back and forth from the elbow joint, as shown.

Breathing: Rhythmically.
Reps: Alternate arm movements until each arm is bent and extended 12 times.

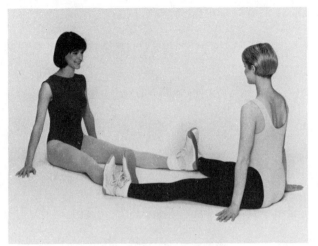 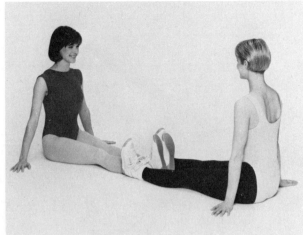

SERIES 2—STATION 1

Straight Leg Adduction
(works inner and outer thighs)

Sit facing your partner, with a straight back, and extend your legs, knees bent and feet flexed. Open your legs and place your feet outside your partner's, as shown. Squeeze your legs together with your inner thighs as your partner resists with her outer thighs. Release the tension and open back to the starting position.

Breathing: Exhale as the legs come together, inhale as the legs release and open.

Reps: 15 times; then exchange positions with your partner.

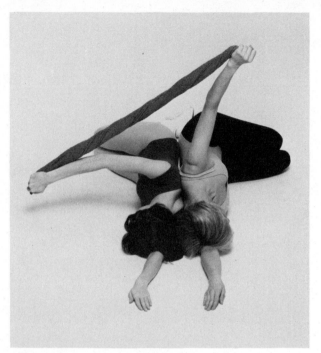 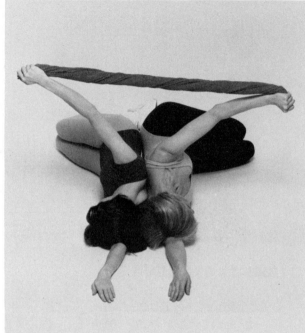

SERIES 2—STATION 2

Lying Cable Pull
(works pectorals and deltoids)

Lie on your side, back to back, as shown. Bend your legs from the hip and knee. One partner extends her working arm up perpendicular to the floor, elbows slightly bent. The other partner extends her working arm in front of her body, elbow bent. Stretch one towel between the two working arms. The partner with the arm extended up, slowly brings her arm down to the floor in front of her chest. The other partner creates smooth resistance by pulling in the opposite direction until her arm is extended directly above her shoulder.

Breathing: Exhale as the hand is brought to the floor, inhale as the hand extends above.

Reps: Each partner should bring the working arm to the floor 12 times.

Note: This is a shoulder joint isolation. Be careful not to bend elbows too much or it will become a bicep exercise.

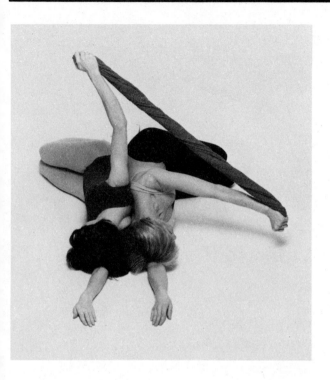

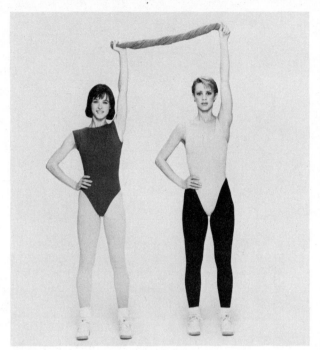
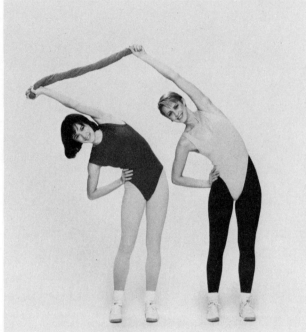

SERIES 2—STATION 3

Sidebend
(works waist)

Stand side by side about a foot and a half apart. Place the right hand on the hip and extend the left arm straight up overhead, as shown. Maintaining tension between the towel held with the hand of the extended arm, bend to the right side. Return back to an upright position and repeat. Resistance is created in both directions.

Breathing: Exhale as you bend to the side, inhale as you return to starting position.

Reps: Bend 15 times to the left side; then change arms and bend 15 times to the right side.

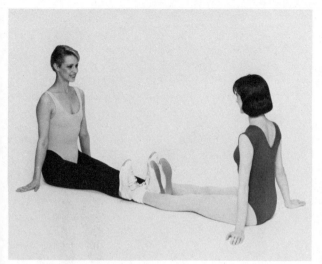 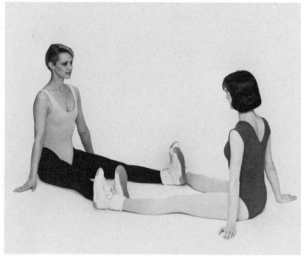

SERIES 2—STATION 4

Straight Leg Abduction
(works inner and outer thighs)

This exercise is performed in a manner similar to Series 2— Station 1 described in this chapter. This time, start with your legs together and extend to an open position.

Breathing: Exhale as you open the legs, inhale as you return to center.
Reps: 15 times; then exchange positions with your partner.

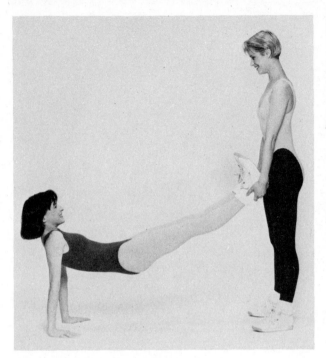
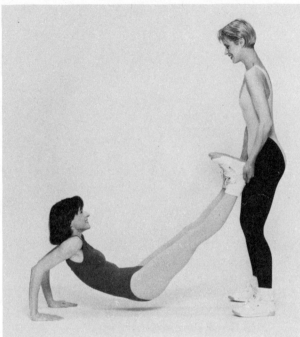

SERIES 2—STATION 5

Elbow Dip
(works tricep)

Sit on the floor, legs extended, hands placed under your shoulders, fingers pointed toward your feet. As your partner picks your feet up, straighten your arms and stretch your body out. To exercise the tricep, bend your elbows and lower the hips. The assisting partner should bend her knees slightly to avoid strain on the lower back. Straighten your arms and repeat.

Breathing: Inhale as you bend the arms, exhale as you straighten the arms.
Reps: 15 times; then exchange places with your partner.

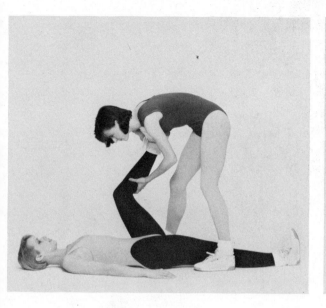
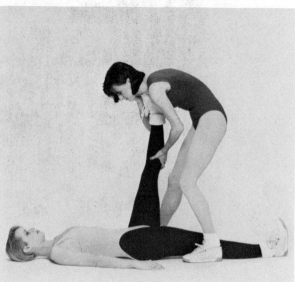

SERIES 3—STATION 1

Leg Press
(works hip and thigh)

Lie on your back, arms by your side. One leg is extended directly under your body; the other leg is extended up, knee bent. Bending over, the assisting partner straddles your body, placing your foot onto her shoulder joints. Her hands are used for additional support, as shown. Your partner creates resistance by pressing down on your foot as you extend your leg to a full 90° position. When the leg is fully extended, release the pressure and return to starting position.

Breathing: Exhale while extending the leg, inhale while lowering the leg.
Reps: 12 times for each leg; then exchange places with your partner.

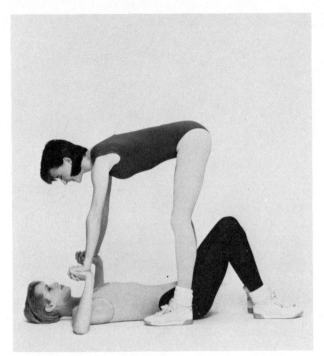
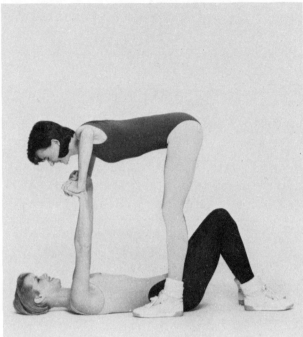

SERIES 3—STATION 2

Partner Push-up
(works pectorals)

Lie on your back, knees bent, feet flat on the floor. Place your elbows at right angles to your body, with your forearms perpendicular to the floor. The assisting partner straddles your hips, bends from her own hips, and, keeping a straight back, reaches down to clasp your hands, as shown. A simultaneous push-up is created when you extend your arms up, pressing against your partner's bending arms. When your arms are fully extended, your partner presses your arms back down while you provide the resistance.

Breathing: Exhale as you extend the arms, inhale as you bend the arms.
Reps: Press up 10 times; then exchange places with your partner.

Note: The standing partner must isolate the shoulders, making sure not to move the back from its perpendicular position.

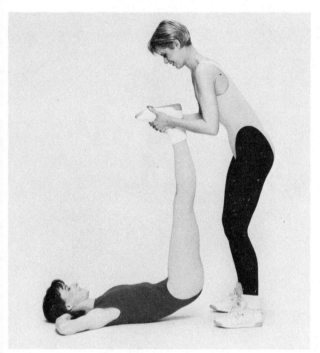 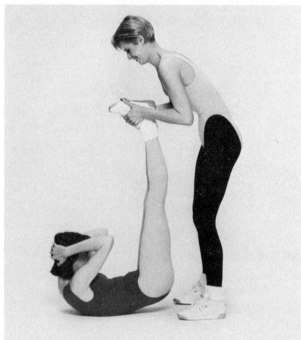

SERIES 3—STATION 3

Isolated Upper Abdominal "Crunch"
(works abdomen)

Lie on your back, legs extended 90° to your body. Lace the fingers behind your head. The assisting partner stands facing your legs. Placing her hands under your feet, she lifts your pelvis off the floor. With your pelvis lifted, bring the elbows together and lift up off your shoulder blades. Return the head and shoulders to the floor and repeat.

Breathing: Exhale as you lift, inhale as you lower.
Reps: 20 times; then exchange places with your partner.

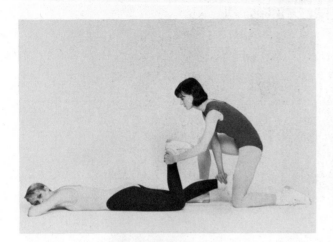 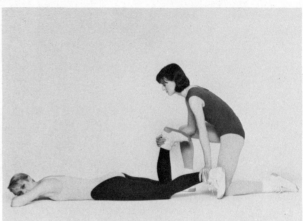

SERIES 3—STATION 4

Alternating Leg Curls
(works hamstrings)

Lie on your abdomen and fold your forearms under your head. To begin
the exercise, lift one leg from the knee joint and keep the other leg
extended. Flex both feet. The assisting partner kneels behind you, placing
her hands on the back of your ankles. Alternate curling your legs from the
knee joint toward the lower back as your partner provides resistance.

Breathing: Rhythmically.
Reps: 12 curls per leg; then exchange places with your partner.

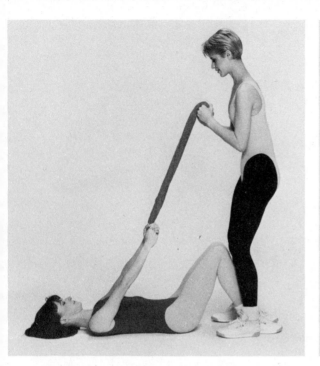 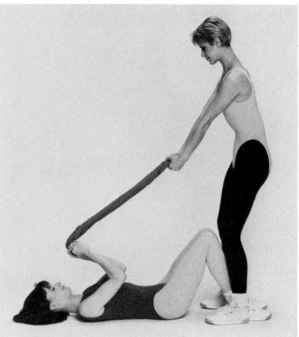

SERIES 3—STATION 5

Isolated Bicep Curls
(works biceps)

Lie on your back, knees bent, feet flat on the floor. Holding one end of a towel, extend your arms at a 45° angle. Straddling your feet, your partner stands over you, holding the other end of the towel, also at a 45° angle but with elbows bent. Maintaining resistance between the towel, alternate curling the forearms back and forth, isolating the shoulder joints.

Breathing: Inhale as you extend, exhale as you curl.
Reps: Alternate a total of 24 curls.

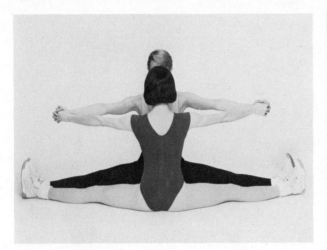 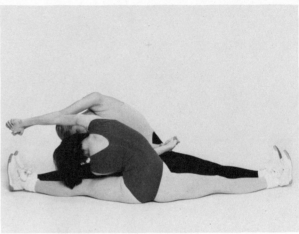

POST-ROUTINE STRETCH #1

Sitting Straddle Stretch
(works hamstrings, inner thighs, waist, shoulders, and arms)

Sit facing each other, with legs open in a wide straddle, feet braced together and with arms extended, fingers laced together, as shown. Bend to the left, bringing the top arms overhead and the bottom arms under toward the opposite legs. Return to starting position and repeat to the other side.

Breathing: Exhale as you bend, inhale as you return to center.
Reps: Alternate sides 6 times, holding end position for 10 seconds.

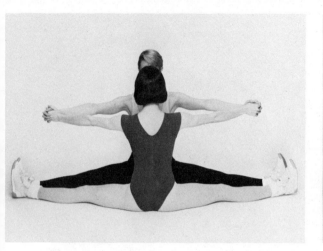 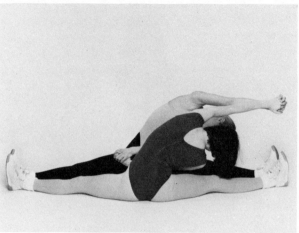

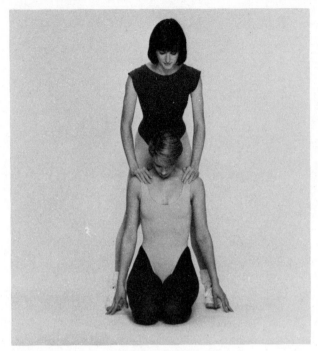
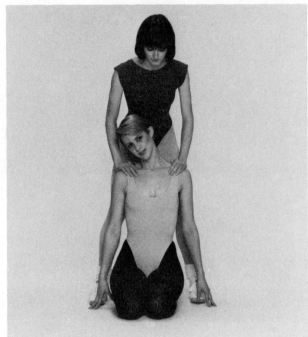

POST-ROUTINE STRETCH #2

Kneeling Neck Circles
(works neck)

Kneel down, sitting on your heels. Stretch your arms down to the floor, keeping a straight back and square shoulders. Your partner should stand behind you, placing her hands on your shoulders to provide resistance. Start by dropping your head forward and rolling to the right, back, left, and return to front.

Breathing: Rhythmically.
Reps: Rotate 4 times in each direction; then exchange places with your partner.

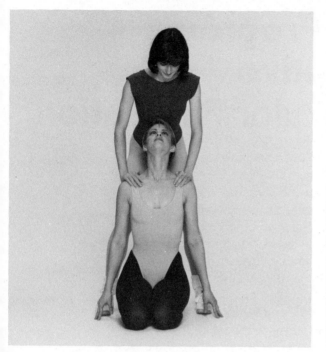
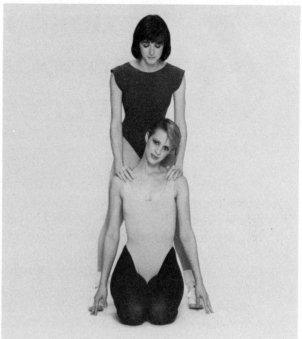

6 Flexibility Program: Proprioceptive Neuromuscular Facilitation

Physiologists refer to two types of stretching, *ballistic* and *static*. Ballistic stretching involves vigorous bouncing movements, as in bobbing down quickly to touch your toes. It was probably the type of stretching you did in grade school class, but we've come a long way in our understanding of exercise physiology since then and now know that instead of intensifying the stretch and bringing faster results, this type of movement actually has the opposite results.

Ballistic stretching activates the *stretch reflex*. The stretch reflex is a neuromuscular feedback mechanism. It is a motor response that activates the reflex contraction of a muscle, which is subject to a pulling force. A familiar example of this complex mechanism is the "knee jerk" test your doctor subjects you to during your annual checkup. He taps the patella tendon, which stretches the neurons within the tendon, and they in turn send a signal to the central nervous system to relay a volley of impulses to the quadriceps (frontal thigh muscles) to contract. The result is that your foot kicks up.

The body uses the stretch reflex in a variety of ways. The stretch reflex protects joints from overextension, and it maintains body equilibrium and posture. The stretch reflex even affects the muscles of the heart. When you begin to exercise, greater volumes of blood are required to supply the muscles in the extremities. The peripheral heart action in the muscles of these extremities forces venous blood back to the heart, which stretches the heart chambers slightly, switching on the "reflex" that speeds the heart to pump even more blood.

Yet another example that will later illuminate our stretching technique is the phenomenon of "stored energy," which is produced by the stretch reflex. When you attempt to swing a racket, bat, or golf club to hit a ball, the motion preceding the follow-through (muscular contraction) is a stretch. This preparatory elongation of the muscle functions to draw more motor units into play, thereby creating more potential strength, that is, stored energy. Another example from daily life is when you walk. Each time you take a step, you stretch your hip flexors (upper thigh muscles). The resulting forward step is partially a reflex contraction, just like the knee-jerk. Later in this chapter, I will show you how we will use this "stored energy" to create greater flexibility. But first, back to the physiology.

All of these stretch reflex reactions happen because of yet another complex physiological mechanism called *proprioception*. Proprioception is the body's ability to sense itself and its relationship to the environment. Even blindfolded, you can tell you are walking up a hill. This awareness is made possible by tiny internal measuring devices that read body position, change of position, rate of change, tension, and loading of resistance. These tiny devices are called proprioceptors, and the body has several types, but the two we are concerned with here are the *muscle spindles* and the *Golgi tendons*.

The muscle spindle's perceiving function is to measure the degree to which a muscle is being stretched *and* the rate or speed at which it is being stretched. Its response function is to tell the muscles to contract. The Golgi tendon's function is also to respond and regulate work stress (stretch and tension), but its response is to make the muscles relax. So it is these two proprioceptors that can protect you from the potentially harmful effects of ballistic stretching.

Ballistic stretching can damage ligaments, tendons, and muscles and result in small muscle tears, which form scars in the tissue. Once formed, the scars are there to stay; they are inelastic and can interrupt blood flow and nerve input and can interfere with subsequent exercise. The proprioceptive stretch reflex tries to prevent these injuries by sending a signal to the brain to reflexively contract the muscles involved in the repetitive, quick bouncing motion of the ballistic stretch. This is also why you get "tight" after the quick repetitive motion of exercise forms such as running, cycling, skiing, and so on, and why you need to stretch out these muscles slowly afterward.

The kind of stretching you should do before and after any intense muscle activity is *static stretching*. Static stretching is not rough or painful, but slow, gentle, and delicate, like the fluid movements of a cat. The static stretching exercises should be done in a slow, thoughtful, gentle manner and should be carefully coordinated with breathing.

If you do not pay attention to your body's magnificent warning system, and you stretch and bounce too far, the stretch reflex causes muscle spasms by packing the injured muscle area with swollen cells, which act as hydraulic splints to prevent any additional movement until the area can heal itself. We have all been laid up with a stiff back from trying to lift something heavy too quickly. The Flexibility Program will teach you to become sensitive to your own stretch reflex response so that you can avoid back injuries.

The Flexibility Program I have devised utilizes a therapeutic technique called *Proprioceptive Neuromuscular Facilitation* (PNF). Simply put, this is the controlled manipulation of the proprioceptive devices. It works by "fooling them" into thinking they are recording a potentially harmful situation and then carefully capitalizes on the neuromuscular responses of relaxation and contraction to attain greater flexibility. This technique is used by physical therapists to release muscle spasms. The program I have designed is a unique application of this method. Following it religiously you will achieve great flexibility gains.

The "superstretch," or PNF method, is effective for two reasons. First, the technique "deinhibits," or reprograms, the stretch reflex, which would ordinarily tell the "tight" muscles to splint to protect carelessly exercised or overused muscles. Second, by practicing the PNF technique regularly, you will create a whole new range of motion within your body joints, a flexibility you may have not thought possible. And, as already stated in our discussion of the physiology and interdependence of the Four Conditioning Components, this increased range of motion can function to prevent injury, create strength, and provide you with the means to perform at a higher level of skill.

PROPRIOCEPTIVE NEUROMUSCULAR FACILITATION

Before attempting these flexibility exercises, you should have a thorough knowledge of the Basic Program (Chapter 4). A thorough warm-up of at least 10 minutes is imperative before you begin this program. There are 14 exercises in this program, covering every major muscle group in sequential order. If your goal is overall body flexibility, this program can be done as often as every day. But even doing it 3 times a week on alternating days for 8 to 12 weeks will give you marked results. In combination with the Basic and Aerobic Programs, add the PNF Program one day, preferably at the end of your workout week. Every exercise in this section uses the following four-step procedure:

1. Both partners place themselves in the appropriate body configurations. With assistance from your partner, *stretch* the muscle(s) to their maximum range of motion. Be sure to exhale with the stretch.
2. Maintaining the stretched position, *contract* the muscles involved against your partner's isometric (nonmovable) resistance for 6 seconds. (Have your partner count out the time.) Exhale with this contraction. Be sure to isolate the body part involved. Do not tense other muscles when you are contracting.
3. *Release* the contraction, but do not move from the stretch position.
4. With assistance from your partner, *stretch* to the newly created range of motion that will result from the "rebound effect" of the isometric contraction. Maintain this new position and repeat *contraction, release, stretch* sequence 3 more times, making a total of 4 stretches and contractions.

After 4 repetitions of the sequence, the muscles and connective tissue reach their fullest "stretch curve."

After you are thoroughly familiar with this technique, you can pick out specific exercises for trouble areas you might have and add them to the end of your existing routines or sports activity.

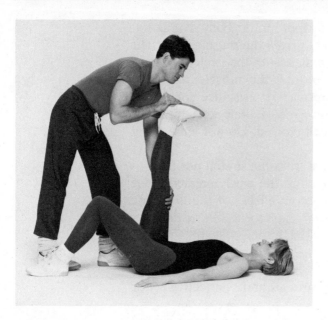

PNF #1

Hamstrings

One partner lies on her back, extending the right leg straight up 90° to the floor, flexing the right foot. Keep this leg as straight as possible. Bending the left leg, place the left foot flat on the floor. Extend the arms comfortably to the side and press the lower back and chin down. The assisting partner stands to the right of your body, placing his right hand on the back of your foot and the left hand just above the knee joint.

1. With assistance from your partner, stretch the extended leg back toward your torso until you feel a *slight* discomfort. Be sure to keep the lower back on the floor.
2. Contract the leg back away from your torso against your partner's isometric (nonmovable) resistance.
3. Release the contraction, but maintain the stretch.
4. Repeat steps 1, 2, and 3 a total of 4 times and work the left leg; then exchange places with your partner.

Breathing: Exhale during the stretches and contractions.

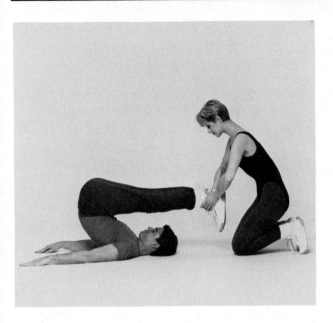

PNF #2

Back and Hamstrings

Lie on your back, roll up onto your shoulders and extend your legs overhead parallel to the floor. Keep your knees straight and your feet flexed. The assisting partner kneels behind you, placing her hands on your ankles.

1. Keeping the legs stationary, stretch your back by rolling down your spine toward your pelvis.
2. Hold that stretch and press your legs up evenly against your partner's hands.
3. Release tension but maintain stretch.
4. Repeat steps 1, 2, and 3 a total of 4 times; then exchange places with your partner.

Breathing: Exhale during the stretches and contractions.

Caution: Be careful not to place too much pressure on the back of your neck.

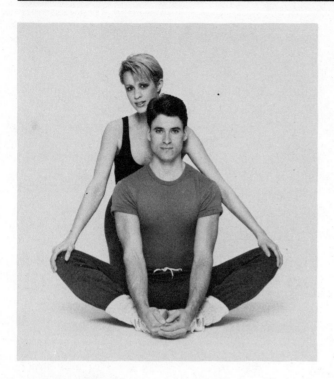

PNF #3

Hips and Inner Thighs

One partner sits down, bends the knees, and opens the legs, placing the soles of the feet together. Clasp your feet with your hands. The assisting partner kneels behind, reaches over your shoulders and places one hand on either knee.

1. With assistance from your partner, stretch your knees down toward the floor.
2. Contract the legs up against your partner's hands.
3. Release the contraction but maintain the stretch.
4. Repeat steps 1, 2, and 3, a total of 4 times; then exchange places with your partner.

Breathing: Exhale during the stretches and contractions.

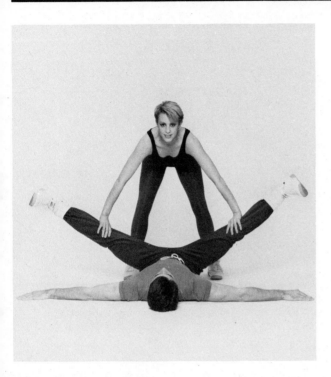

PNF #4

Inner Thighs

Lie on your back, extend your legs out to the side 90° to your body.
Stretch your arms comfortably out to the sides of your body and press
your chin down. The assisting partner stands facing you, placing her
hands on your inner thighs, as shown.

1. Stretch the legs toward the floor with pressure from your partner.
2. Maintain that increased stretch position and contract against your
   partner's stationary hands.
3. Release the contraction but maintain stretch.
4. Repeat steps 1, 2, and 3 a total of 4 times; then exchange places with
   your partner.

Breathing: Exhale during the stretches and contractions.

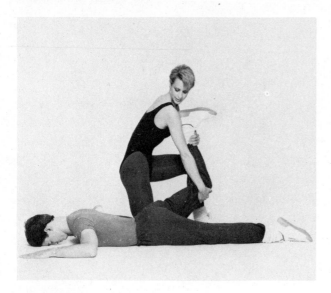

PNF #5

Quadriceps—Front Thigh

Lie on your stomach, placing your forehead on the floor, bringing your forearms up and parallel to your head, as shown. Lift the right leg straight up. The assisting partner kneels at your right side, placing her right hand under your right knee and placing the left hand under the foot.

1. The thigh is stretched with assistance from your partner by lifting the leg up, keeping the knee bent.
2. Maintaining this increased stretch, press your thigh back down against your partner's stationary resistance.
3. Release the pressure of the contraction but maintain stretch.
4. Repeat steps 1, 2, and 3 a total of 4 times for each leg; then exchange places with your partner.

Breathing: Exhale during the stretches and contractions.

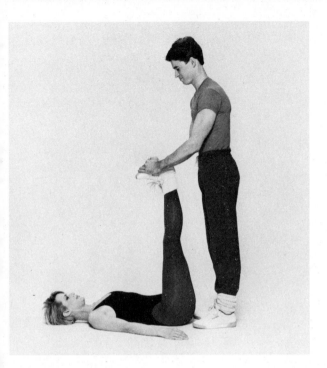

PNF #6

Achilles and Calves

One partner lies on the back, legs extended straight up 90° to the floor and arms stretched comfortably down by the side, chin down. The assisting partner stands to the back of the legs and places one hand on each foot.

1. Keeping the legs stationary, stretch the feet back toward your body with pressure from your partner.
2. Maintain increased stretch and contract against your partner's stationary hands.
3. Release pressure but maintain stretch.
4. Repeat steps 1, 2, and 3 a total of 4 times; then exchange positions with your partner.

Breathing: Exhale during the stretches and contractions.

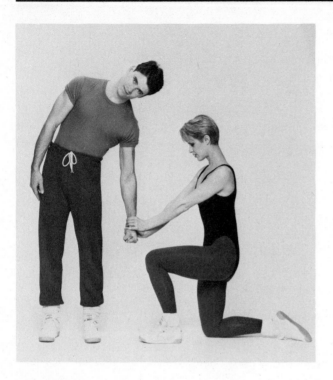

PNF #7

Obliques (Waist)

One partner stands, legs parallel, feet at hip width apart. Bend over to the left side. Let your neck relax. The assisting partner kneels next to you, clasping both hands around your wrists, as shown.

1. Stretch down toward the floor with assistance from your partner.
2. Maintaining increased stretch, try to pull back up toward an upright position against your partner's stationary resistance.
3. Release contraction but maintain stretch.
4. Repeat steps 1, 2, and 3 a total of 4 times per side; then exchange positions with your partner.

Breathing: Exhale during the stretches and contractions.

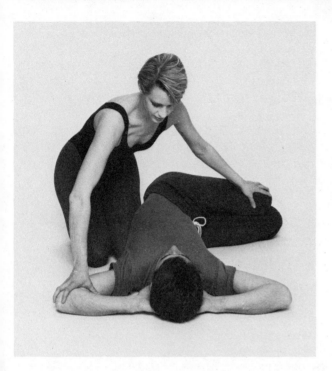

PNF #8

Lower Back, Buttocks, Outside Thighs, Chest, and Arms

Lie on your back, bend the knees, and twist them to the right side 90° to the body, as shown. Lace the fingers behind the back of your head, pressing the elbows down to the floor. The assisting partner kneels to your left side, placing her right hand on your left elbow and her left hand on your left knee.

1. Downward pressure is applied by your partner on the elbow and knee to create the stretch.
2. Pressing up against your partner's hands, contract the muscles involved.
3. Release the stationary contraction, still maintaining the stretch.
4. Repeat steps 1, 2, and 3 a total of 4 times for both sides of the body; then exchange places with your partner.

Breathing: Exhale during the stretches and contractions.

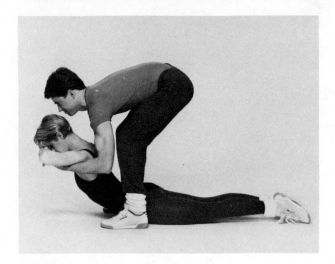

PNF #9

Stomach and Chest

One partner lies face down, lacing the fingers together under the forehead. Keep legs together. The assisting partner squats over your back, places his hands under your bent arms and gently lifts your torso.

1. Partner lifts you to a comfortable height.
2. Press your torso down toward the floor against your partner's hands.
3. Release the tension momentarily but maintain stretch.
4. Repeat steps 1, 2, and 3 a total of 4 times; then exchange places with your partner.

Breathing: Exhale during the stretches and contractions.

Caution: People with bad lower backs should do this exercise cautiously.

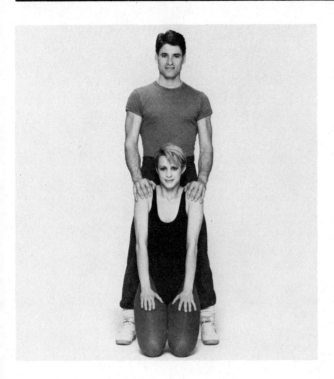

PNF #10

Trapezius and Shoulders

Kneel down, legs together, sitting on your heels. Place your hands on your thighs. Your partner stands behind you, placing his hands on your shoulders, as shown.

1. Stretch your shoulders straight down toward the floor.
2. Shrug the shoulders upward against your partner's isometric (nonmovable) resistance.
3. Relax the contraction, but maintain stretch.
4. Repeat steps 1, 2, and 3 a total of 4 times; then exchange places with your partner.

Breathing: Exhale during the stretches and contractions.

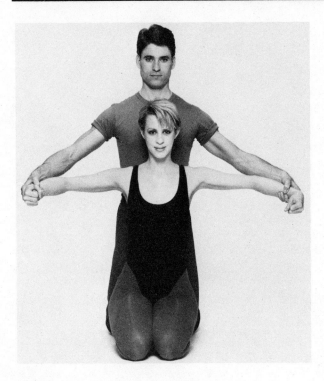

PNF #11

Chest and Shoulders

One partner kneels down on the floor, legs together, sitting on her heels. Keep the head and chest erect. Stretch your arms back behind your body, parallel to the floor, as shown. Arms slightly bent. The assisting partner kneels behind, clasping each wrist.

1. The assisting partner stretches your arms backward until you feel a *slight* discomfort.
2. Press the bent arms forward against your partner's isometric (nonmovable) resistance.
3. Release contraction, but maintain stretch.
4. Repeat steps 1, 2, and 3 a total of 4 times; then exchange places with your partner.

Breathing: Exhale during the stretches and contractions.

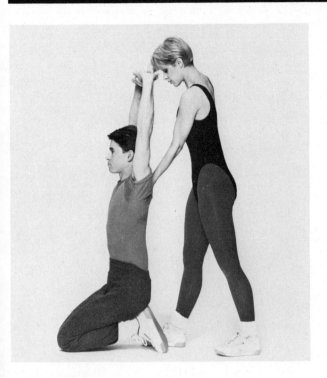

PNF #12

Shoulders and Triceps

Kneel in the same position as in exercise #11, except lace the fingers together; extend the arms overhead, palms facing up, as shown. The assisting partner places one hand between the shoulder blades and the other hand in front of your clasped hands.

1. With help from your partner, stretch the arms back from your shoulder joints (not from the lower back).
2. Press the arms forward against your partner's resistance.
3. Release the contraction but maintain the stretch.
4. Repeat steps 1, 2, and 3 a total of 4 times; then exchange places with your partner.

Breathing: Exhale during the stretches and contractions.

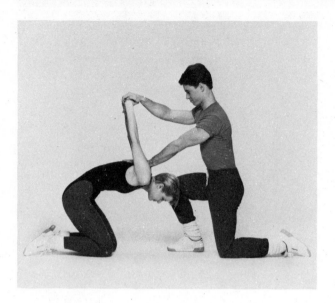

PNF #13

Shoulders and Biceps

One partner kneels down, legs together. Lace the fingers together behind your back and lift the arms up toward your head, bending over from the waist at the same time. As in exercise #12, your partner places one hand between your shoulders, but the other hand is behind your clasped hands.

1. With assistance, gently stretch your arms forward from the shoulder joints, keeping the arms straight. Keep neck muscles relaxed.
2. Press your hands back toward your pelvis, against your partner's nonmovable resistance. Do not move from the waist.
3. Release contraction but maintain stretch.
4. Repeat steps 1, 2, and 3 a total of 4 times; then exchange places with your partner.

Breathing: Exhale during the stretches and contractions.

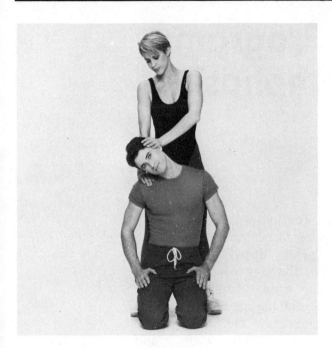

PNF #14

Neck

Kneel down, sitting on your heels, resting your hands on your thighs. Comfortably stretch your head to one side, keeping your shoulders and back stable. The assisting partner should stand behind you, placing one hand on your shoulder and the other hand on the side of your head, as shown.

1. Have your partner provide additional pressure, stretching the neck in the direction that the head is tilted.
2. Press your head against your partner's hand (toward the stretching muscle).
3. Release contraction but maintain stretch.
4. Repeat steps 1, 2, and 3 a total of 4 times for each direction: right, left, forward, backward. (In the forward position, partner's hands should be placed on the back of the head; in the backward position, the partner's hand is placed on the forehead); then exchange places with your partner.

Breathing: Exhale during the stretches and contractions.

7 Advanced Program: Negative Emphasis Training

While the movement principles Continuous Tension and Peak Contraction in the Basic Program (Chapter 4) increase *muscular endurance*, the movement principle of Negative Emphasis develops "strength per contraction," or *force*. As with the Basic Program, the goal of the Negative Emphasis Training Program is to fire as many muscle fibers as possible and to bring those fibers up to maximum contractile capacity. But with Negative Emphasis Training, you will be increasing the width of the muscle as well. This increase in muscle size is known as *hypertrophy*, and it is brought about by increasing the amount of connective tissue and the number of microscopic protein filaments and blood capillaries. Simply put, this program of Negative Emphasis Training develops muscle size, more size means more strength, and, conversely, more strength provides the means to create more size.

Developing this type of muscle strength is desirable if you have a job that requires lifting or pushing, or if you play a sport that requires pushing and blocking, like football, or if you just want to redefine your shape by increasing inches in the width of your back or in the size of your arms.

In performing these exercises, you should keep in mind that you can only "spot increase" a body part; you can't "spot reduce" a body part. This is because muscle tissue behaves differently from adipose (fat) tissue. You are born with a certain number of fat cells, and you more or less retain this number throughout your life, regardless of how many pounds you may gain or lose. When you gain fat, you are not increasing the number of fat cells, but are making the ones you have bigger, and likewise, when you lose fat, you are not actually losing fat cells but are shrinking the size of the ones you have. Fat cells shrink or gain in size all at the same time, but the body's muscle tissue *does* respond to localized attention, which makes it possible to isolate muscle tissue growth.

To explain how Negative Emphasis Training works, we need to look at two phases of muscle contraction. There is the *positive* or *concentric* phase, in which the muscle shortens as it does its work, and the *negative* or *eccentric* phase, in which the muscle lengthens as it does its work. Studies show that when a muscle is in the eccentric, or lengthening, phase, it can handle more resistance than when it is shortening. We've all experienced how much easier it is to lower a heavy object than it is to lift it. Muscles lengthen when they work with gravity and shorten when they work against gravity.

When you increase your capacity to handle greater work overloads by working negatively, you will achieve greater increases in muscle strength and size. In this program, you will achieve this "additional resistance" with your partner by moving only through the negative phase of the movement and/or by working one body part against two.

This effective strength and size-building program must be used intelligently because it is easy to overtrain with this Negative Emphasis method. Microscopic tears within the muscle fibers are a normal by-product of any resistance training because the contractile fibers are lengthening to their full capacity while they are doing the work. These tears are partially responsible for the muscle soreness that occurs the day after a workout. I recommend that you perform these exercises sensibly and combine them with exercises in the Flexibility Program (Chapter 6) to help alleviate the additional soreness.

NEGATIVE EMPHASIS TRAINING

The Negative Emphasis Training Program consists of the following:

- 4 additional warm-up exercises:
  2 pre-routine abdomen exercises
  2 pre-routine flexibility exercises
- 2 lower body exercises
- 8 upper body exercises
- 2 post-routine abdomen exercises
- 3 post-routine flexibility exercises

Because of the additional soreness resulting from these exercises, I recommend this program for 1 or 2 nonconsecutive days per week. You should be completely familiar with the Basic Program (Chapter 4) before attempting this program.

In combination with the other programs, try the following schedules:

1. Basic: 2 times per week (Mon., Wed.)
   Negative: 1 time (Fri.)
2. Negative: 2 times per week (Mon., Wed.)
   PNF: 1 time (Fri.)
3. Basic: 2 times per week (Mon., Wed.)
   ACT/PHA: 2 times per week (Tues., Thurs.)
   Negative: 1 time (Fri.)
   PNF: 1 time (Sat.)

You should warm up for 5 to 10 minutes. Leave no more than 2 minutes between exercises, but do not rush. In this technique, the breathing is done opposite—the exhalation is on the eccentric contraction rather than on the concentric contraction as in the Basic Program. This is because a maximal effort is exerted on the eccentric contraction only. See specific breathing instructions in each exercise. Maximum effort should be exerted with each rep. Maintain *strict* form and remember to cooperate, not compete.

Once you are familiar with this technique, you can incorporate individual exercises in other programs to increase strength or to shape a specific body part.

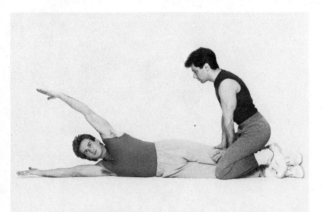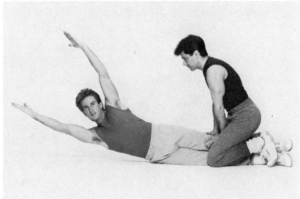

PRE-ROUTINE AB EXERCISE #1

Straight Body—Oblique Lift
(strengthens abdomen)

Lie on your side, legs together, arms outstretched overhead. The assisting partner straddles your legs in a kneeling position and holds your legs down, as shown. In a quick, two-count motion, lift the entire torso up to the hip. Lower the torso and arms in a slow four-count motion.

Breathing: Exhale as you lift, inhale as you lower.
Reps: 25 times and change sides; then exchange places with your partner.

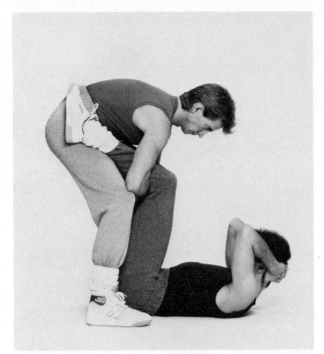 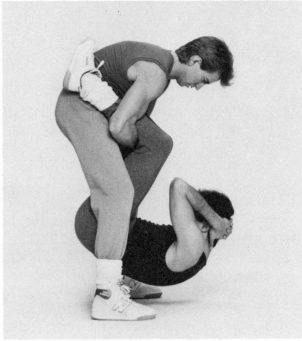

PRE-ROUTINE AB EXERCISE #2

Antigravitational "Crunch"
(strengthens abdomen and hip flexors)

Lie on your back and lace your fingers behind your head, with elbows
chest width apart. The assisting partner straddles your hips in a bent hip/
bent-knee position, as shown. He locks his forearms under your knees,
while you wrap your feet around his hips. As you bring your elbows
toward your knees, your partner simultaneously lifts his back slightly so
that you rise completely off the floor. Lower back down in a slow four-
count motion.

Breathing: Exhale as you rise, inhale as you lower.
Reps: As many times as you can; then exchange places with your partner.

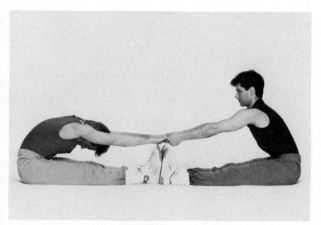 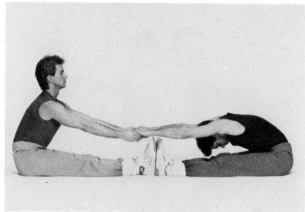

PRE-ROUTINE STRETCH #1

Sitting Pull
(works hamstrings, back, and arms)

Sit facing your partner, legs extended, soles of the feet braced together. Reach forward, clasping your partner's hands and simultaneously stretch forward as your partner pulls backward in alternating stretches.

Breathing: Exhale as you reach forward, inhale as you go backward.
Reps: 6 forward stretches, each held for 10 seconds.

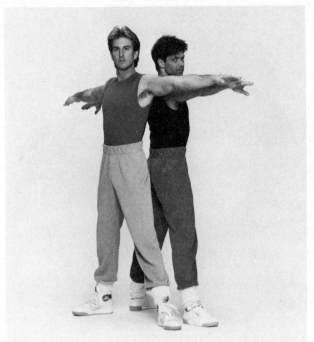 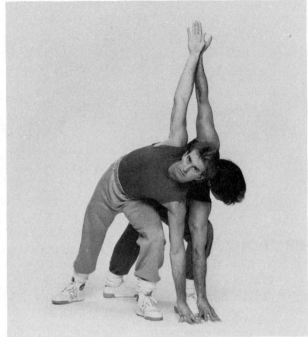

PRE-ROUTINE STRETCH #2

Side Lunge
(works hamstrings, inner thighs, arms, and obliques)

Stand back to back, about 6 inches apart. Open the legs 2 feet, turn the front foot forward, and the back foot out, as shown. Stretch the arms out parallel to the floor. Using your partner for balance, lunge forward, bending your front leg and keeping your back leg straight until your forward hand reaches the floor. Arms remain perpendicular to the body. Return to starting position and repeat.

Breathing: Exhale as you lunge, inhale as you return to starting position.
Reps: Repeat 4 times and then lunge to the other side. Hold each lunge for 10 seconds.

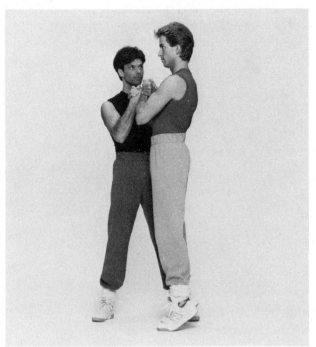 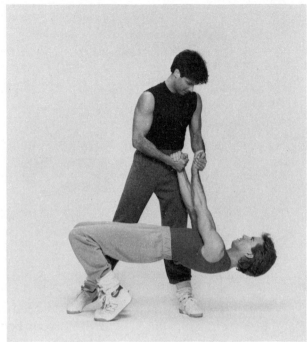

Sissy Squats
(strengthens quadriceps)

Both partners begin by standing at a right angle to one another. The assisting partner's legs are open, while you stand on the balls of your feet, legs 6 inches apart. Clasp your hands tightly and cross wrists. Simultaneously extend your arms, bend your knees, and slowly lower your body, keeping a straight line from the top of the head through the knees, as shown. Do not arch the back or neck. The assisting partner then lifts you back to the starting position.

Breathing: Exhale as you lower, inhale as you rise.
Reps: 20 times; then exchange places with your partner.

Note: The assisting partner exercises his arms and upper back.

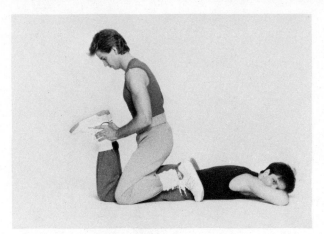 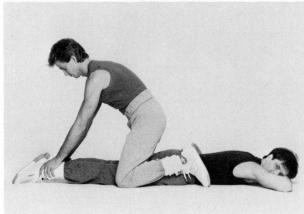

Hamstring Curls
(strengthens hamstrings)

Lie on your abdomen, legs together, head resting on your folded arms. Begin with your knees bent 90° to your body. Your partner straddles your legs in a kneeling position, places his hands on your ankles and slowly presses your feet to the floor in 4 counts. Release back to starting position.

Breathing: Exhale as the legs extend, inhale on the release.
Reps: 20 times; then exchange places with your partner.

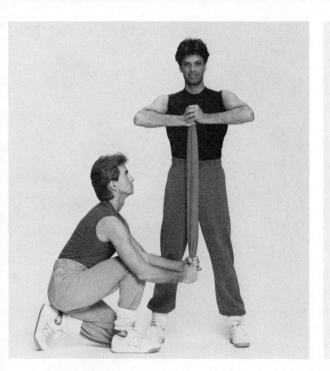 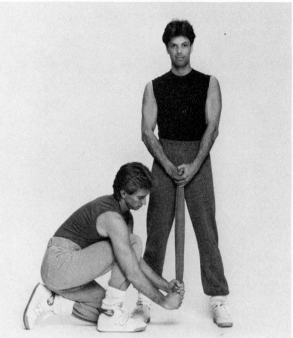

Upright Row
(strengthens trapezius and deltoids)

Stand with your legs open, clasping a towel with two hands, as shown. Your elbows should be lifted parallel to the floor. The assisting partner kneels next to you, holding the other end of the towel. The exercise is done by the assisting partner pulling straight down with the towel until your arms are straight. The resistance is in one direction only—down. Release back up to starting position and repeat.

Breathing: Exhale as the arms go down, inhale on the way up.
Reps: 12 times; then exchange places with your partner.

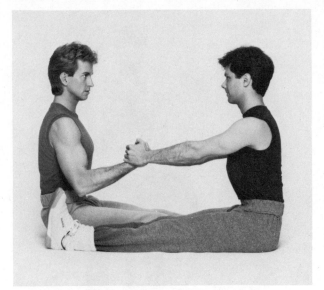 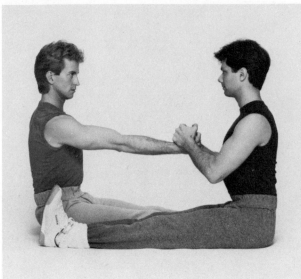

One Arm "Lat" Pull
(strengthens latissimus dorsi)

Sit directly next to your partner, legs extended, knees straight, feet flexed, lower back lifted. You will be working one arm at a time. Your partner will clasp both hands around your wrists and fists. Start from a bent-arm position, elbow by your side. In four counts, your partner will slowly pull with both of his hands on your fist until your bent arm is fully extended. Release the tension back to the bent-arm position and repeat.

Breathing: Exhale as the arm is extended, inhale on the release.
Reps: 12 times per arm; then exchange assisting roles.

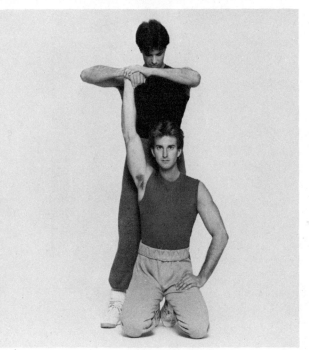 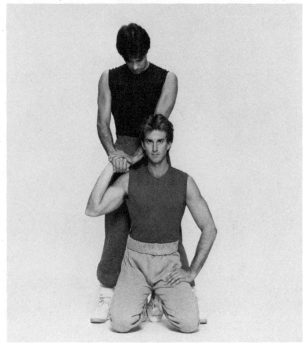

One Arm Military Press
(strengthens deltoid and triceps)

Facing the same direction, one partner kneels down, sitting on his heels, while the assisting partner stands behind. Begin by extending one arm straight up and maintaining an erect spine. The assisting partner clasps two hands on top of your one, as shown, and presses down until your hand has reached your shoulder. Use four counts of smooth, pressured resistance. Release to the top and begin again.

Breathing: Exhale down, inhale up.
Reps: 12 times and change arms; then exchange places with your partner.

Note: Assisting partner gets tricep work.

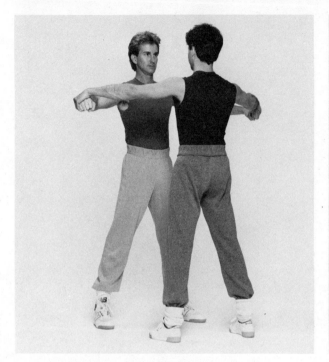
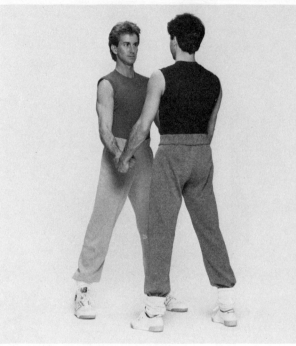

Negative Side Lateral
(strengthens pectorals and deltoids)

Stand squarely, face to face, about 1 foot apart, legs open about 18 inches. This is a dual purpose exercise. Start with your arms raised parallel to the floor, extended slightly in front of your body, elbows slightly bent, with forearms rotated up. The assisting partner puts his arms into the same position but places his hands on top of yours. In a four-count motion, the assisting partner presses the arms down until they are in front of your hips. Release tension and move back to original position. It is important that the movement originates from the shoulders only. Keep the arms fixed. Do not bend the elbow joint. The shoulder joint is the fulcrum, and the arm acts as the lever.

Breathing: Exhale as the arms are lowered, inhale as they release to the top.

Reps: 12 times and change hand positions.

Note: Partner with hands under gets deltoid work, partner with hands on top gets positive contraction pec work.

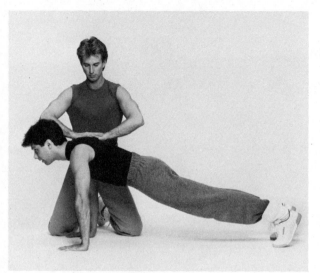 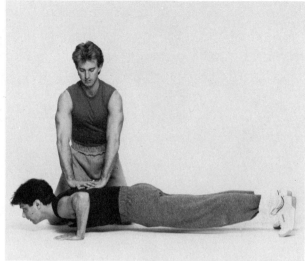

Negative Push-up
(strengthens chest and triceps)

Begin in an upright push-up position, hands and arms pointed in any direction (pick any position from the freebody exercises in Chapter 3). Your partner kneels beside you, as shown, places his hands between your shoulder blades and presses down as you lower your body, resisting the pressure. Release tension and return to starting position.

Breathing: Exhale as you lower, inhale as you return up.
Reps: 12 times; then exchange places with your partner.

Note: Assisting partner gets negative tricep work.

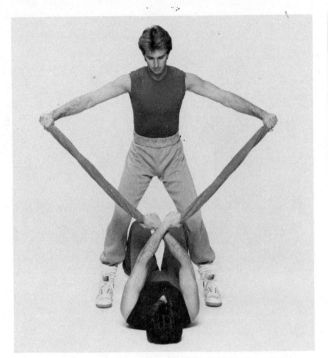 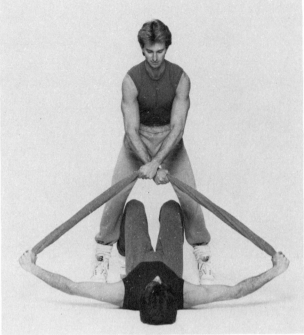

Cross Cable Pull
(strengthens chest, rhomboids, and middle back)

One partner lies on his back, knees bent, wrists crossed, holding the ends of two towels, as shown. The other partner stands, straddling your legs, holding the other ends of the two towels, arms stretched out and open. Both partners' elbows are slightly bent, and the movement is from the shoulder joint. The assisting partner, who is lying down, opens his arms, creating resistance for the standing partner, who slowly brings his arms together until wrists are crossed. Release tension and move arms back to starting position.

Breathing: Exhale as the standing partner's arms come together, inhale as they open.

Reps: 12 times; then exchange places with your partner.

Note: Standing partner gets chest work, lying partner gets middle back work.

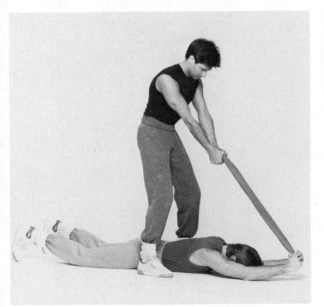 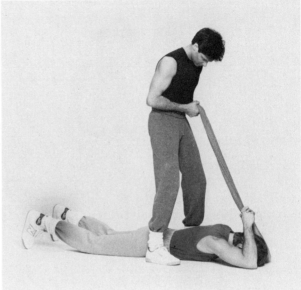

Lying Tricep Extension
(works tricep)

One partner lies face down, legs together, with both hands clasping the end of one towel, as shown. The assisting partner stands, straddling your hips, holding the other end of the towel. Both begin with straight arms. Maintaining tension on the towel, the standing partner pulls from the elbow and shoulder joints, while the lying partner resists by bending the arms from the elbow joints only.

Breathing: Exhale as the arms move forward, inhale as the arms return. Release tension and return to starting position.

Reps: 12 times; then exchange places with your partner.

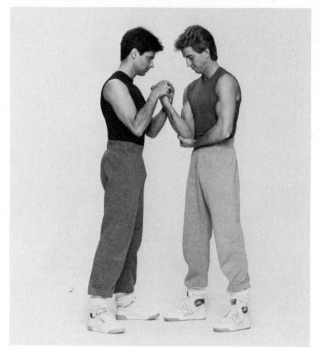 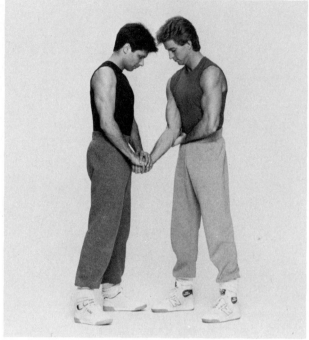

Standing One Arm Curl
(works bicep)

Stand facing one another, at a slight angle. Cup your left hand under your right elbow, which is fully bent and placed close to your side. Make a fist. The assisting partner, placing both hands over your fist, presses down from his elbow joints, until your arm is fully extended. Release and return to starting position.

Breathing: Exhale as the arm is extended, inhale on release.
Reps: 12 times per arm; then exchange places with your partner.

Note: While you are getting negative bicep work, your partner is getting negative tricep work.

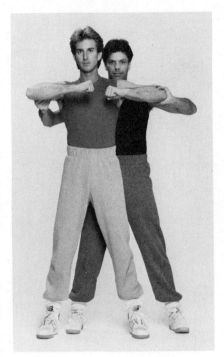
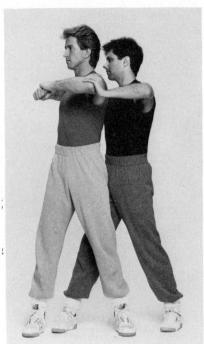
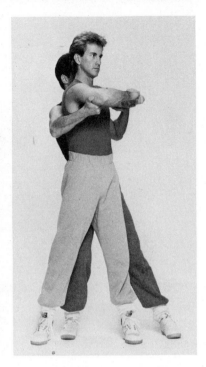

POST-ROUTINE AB EXERCISE #1

Standing Oblique Side Twist
(works waist)

Stand facing the same direction, one in front of the other. The partner in front raises his arms, bending the elbows and bringing the hands together. The other partner places one hand behind your left elbow and the other hand inside your right elbow. Begin the motion by twisting to the right from the hip. Keeping the arms parallel to the floor and isolated in the shoulder and elbow, simultaneously twist the torso through the center until you reach a 90° twist to the left. The partner behind then reverses his hand position, and the twisting movement is repeated to the right.

Breathing: Inhale in preparation for the movement, exhale on the twist.
Reps: 10 times per side; then exchange places with your partner.

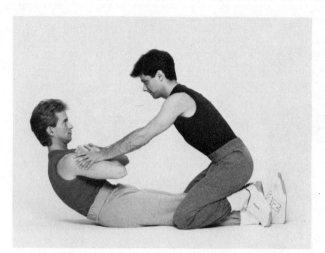
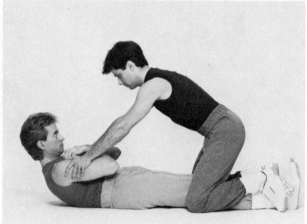

POST-ROUTINE AB EXERCISE #2

Negative Abdominal Press-down
(works upper abdominals)

Lie on your back, legs together, arms folded across the chest. Your partner
kneels down, straddling your knees. Begin in a lifted position, with
shoulders about 1 foot off the floor. The assisting partner places one hand
on each shoulder, as shown. Using his body weight, he presses your torso
toward the floor. Negative pressure is created as you resist your partner's
push. Release tension and raise torso to original height.

Breathing: Exhale on the way down, inhale on the way up.
Reps: 20 times; then exchange places with your partner.

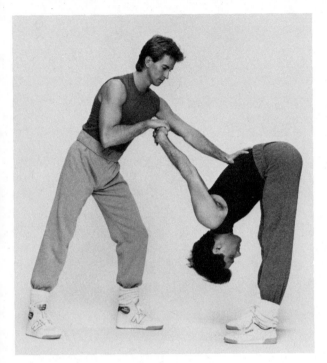 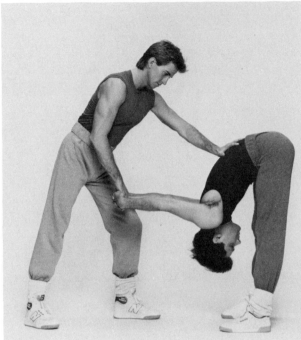

POST-ROUTINE STRETCH #1

Arm Pull-over
(works biceps, shoulders, hamstrings, and back)

Stand with feet one foot apart. Lace your fingers together behind your back and bend over from the waist, extending arms, as shown. The assisting partner places one hand on your lower back and the other hand on the back of your hands, slowly stretching the arms toward the floor. Hold end position for 10 seconds.

Breathing: Exhale as the arms are pulled over, inhale as you return to starting position.

Reps: 6 times; then exchange places with your partner.

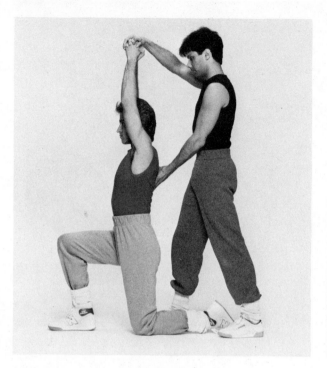 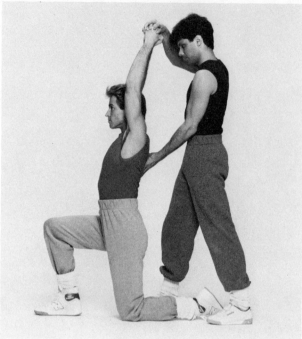

POST-ROUTINE STRETCH #2

Arm Pull-back
(works shoulder, chest, and tricep)

Kneel on your left knee, lifting the right knee and placing the right foot on
the floor. Lace the fingers together directly above your head. The assisting
partner stands behind you, placing his left hand between your shoulder
blades and clasping his right hand over your fist. The stretch is created
when your partner gently pulls your arms back from the shoulder sockets,
not from the lower back.

Breathing: Exhale as the arms are pulled back, inhale on the release.
Reps: 6 times; then exchange places with your partner.

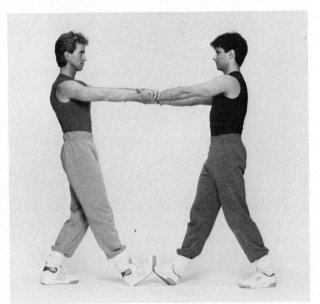 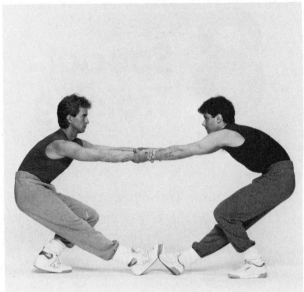

POST-ROUTINE STRETCH #3

Standing "Lat" Pull
(works hamstrings, back, shoulders, and arms)

Stand facing one another, bracing opposite feet together. Clasping each other's wrists, place the other foot about 2 feet behind for balance. Slowly lower yourselves by bending the back knee, keeping the front leg straight, as shown. Keep the arms straight and parallel to the floor. Slowly raise torso up and repeat. Hold bottom position for 10 seconds.

Breathing: Exhale as you lower your body, inhale on the way up.
Reps: Complete 3 stretches per leg.

8 Special Training

The Special Training chapter completes my system and offers you the opportunity to vary your exercises and routines to avoid mental and muscular boredom. This program includes more advanced exercises for various body parts and demonstrates how partners with widely varying body types or fitness levels can work together. Before attempting any of these exercises, you should have thoroughly learned the exercises in the Basic Program (Chapter 4).

Power and Speed. As you become more expert in the partner technique, you may want to experiment with additional training methods. For example, you may be involved in a sport that requires greater speed or power, such as sprinting to first base or hitting a harder tennis serve. In accordance with the specificity principle, you refine a particular motor skill only by practicing that same skill; you improve your tennis serve by practicing your tennis serve. However, you can train a particular muscle or group of muscles to achieve a higher level of speed or power and prepare it for a specific task. This is called working for "special" strength. You can achieve this "special" strength by increasing the speed of movement during the exercise. (Studies show that working at faster speeds with strong resistance engages more muscle fibers.) While working at these accelerated speeds, be sure to maintain smooth, continuous tension throughout the complete range of motion.

Creating Symmetry and Healing Injury. As mentioned in the partner mechanics section (Chapter 2), the partner technique does all that the machines can do and more, including developing body symmetry and rehabilitating injuries. The body has a natural seeking system to create balance, and when there is imbalance, you feel it. If one side of your body is stronger than the other, you can use the exercises in this program to equalize the discrepancy, training the weak, underdeveloped side with additional and stronger repetitions. If you have suffered a localized injury, you do not have to give up training altogether. If you injure one leg, with my technique you can still train the other, and as the injured body part starts to recover, you can start with light pressure and gradually increase the pressure (as long as you feel no pain) and build it back up to its original degree of fitness. You can also rehabilitate an injured area by stretching and strengthening it within a limited range of motion. This will aid in the healing by bringing fresh blood to the area and washing away harmful waste products. Collaborating with renowned doctors, I have used these exercises to rehabilitate patients with serious limb and back injuries, but you should consult a doctor before attempting any rehabilitative exercise.

Of all the techniques of building quick strength and muscle size, I prefer the method of "supersetting," that is, working the agonist muscle, or prime mover, in a particular movement, and then the antagonist, the muscle that offers resistance to the movement, without a rest in between sets. For example, I will do a bicep curl (see Chapter 4), which uses the tricep as the antagonist, and then immediately a tricep extension (see Chapter 4), which conversely uses the bicep as antagonist. You get a great "pump" using this "supersetting" method.

After years of practicing the partner technique, I find that I am creating new exercises all the time, and after a few months of working with the routines, you will begin to see that the variety of exercises you can employ is only limited by your own imagination.

THE SPECIAL TRAINING SECTION

This section is divided by body part, special partner, and flexibility exercises. Some of these exercises are advanced, so be sure to learn the Basic Program (Chapter 4) first.

Use this section to *vary* your routines. When you are first beginning a new training routine or learning a new exercise, the nervous system is usually in a state of excitation and responds with a high energy level, enabling swift, physiological changes. However, after a certain period of time, the nervous system actually becomes stagnated and progress becomes difficult. Muscle boredom sets in. Use the exercises in this section to stimulate your nervous system and add variety to your routines.

Adapt Your Training. If a particular muscle or muscle group feels tired or overworked, or if you have had an injury, don't give up your training. Be adaptable. Work another body part. If you want to work your arms and your partner doesn't, turn to the specific body part section and pick exercises where your partner is providing resistance without working his arms. If your partner wants to work her legs and you don't, pick exercises where you supply the resistance without working your legs.

Be Specific. Look for body part exercises in this section that will help you strengthen muscles used in your particular sport, for example, choosing shoulder exercises to improve your tennis serve. Picking exercises to improve your golf swing will not help you become a better skier.

Always approach your training with intuition. Training is an art and a science. I have provided the scientific means with sophisticated physiology and biomechanics and with prescriptions for days of the week, number of exercises, and so on. You need to apply the art of knowing when to vary, adapt, and specify your routines to meet your individual goals.

BODY PARTS

This section contains 30 exercises for these body parts: abdomen, legs, hips, back, shoulders, chest, and arms.

Abdomen

Most of the abdominal exercises are advanced. Exercise caution. People with bad lower backs should stick to the Basic Ab work. Abdominal exercises can be done every day. The abdominal muscles are "antigravitational" muscles, that is, they aid in maintaining upright posture. To do so, nature has provided the muscle cells with high oxygen-carrying capacity. This means that they are made for endurance and to remove waste products (acids) quickly. So knock yourself out!

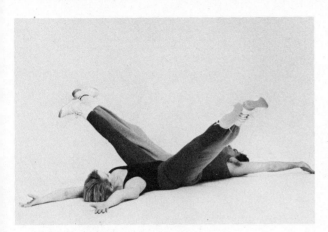 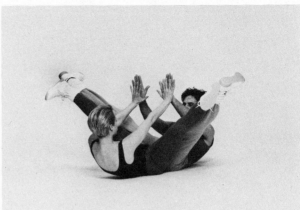

ABDOMEN

Straddle Ab Curl

Lie on your back, facing your partner, legs touching and open in a straddle, as shown. Start with arms stretched back overhead and simultaneously lift your back off the floor and touch hands. Lower back to the floor and repeat.

Breathing: Exhale on the way up, inhale on the way down.
Reps: 20 times.

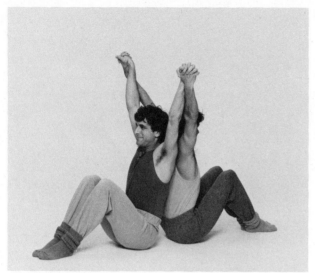 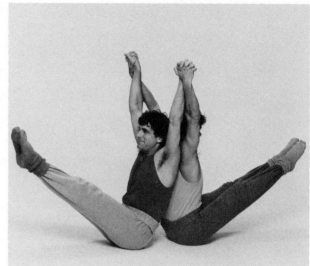

ABDOMEN

Double Leg Extension

Sit back to back, knees bent, extend the arms straight up, and clasp hands. Using your partner's hands for support and balance, simultaneously extend the legs from the knee joint. Feet pointed, bend the knees back to the starting position and repeat.

Breathing: Exhale as you extend, inhale as you bend.
Reps: 20 times.

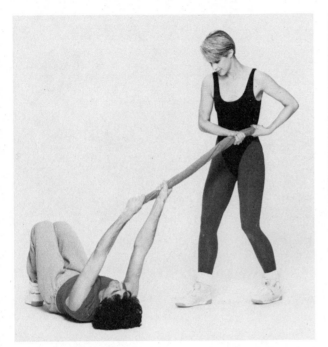
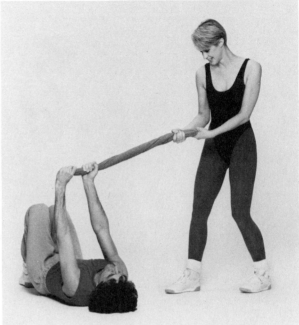

ABDOMEN

Stiff Arm Twisting Pull

Lie on your back, knees bent, arms extended straight over chest, clasping one end of a towel. The assisting partner stands to your side about 3 feet away, holding the other end of the towel. Keeping the shoulders down, begin the exercise by extending your arms to the side and pulling the towel back to center above your chest. Release to the side and repeat. Your partner provides resistance with arm strength and body weight.

Breathing: Exhale as the arms come to the center, inhale on release.
Reps: 15 times per side.

Note: This appears to be a shoulder exercise, but when the arms are kept straight and the spine is pressed down, the abdomen is isolated.

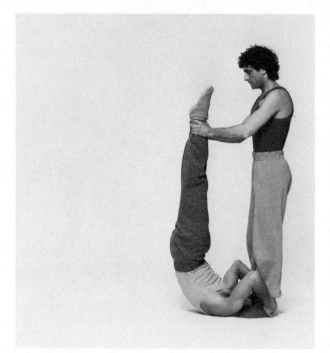 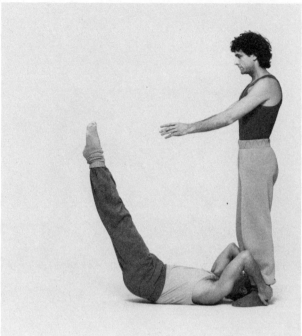

ADVANCED ABDOMEN

Negative Roll-Down

Clasping the ankles of your partner, as shown, begin the exercise by rolling up onto your shoulders, extending your legs, feet pointed, parallel to your partner's standing body. Your partner then grabs your ankles and pushes your legs back down toward the floor, keeping your legs together. Roll down your spine, resisting the momentum of your partner's push, end with feet 1 foot off the floor, and then repeat by rolling back to a shoulder stand.

Breathing: Exhale as you go down, inhale as you roll up.
Reps: 20 times; then exchange places with your partner.

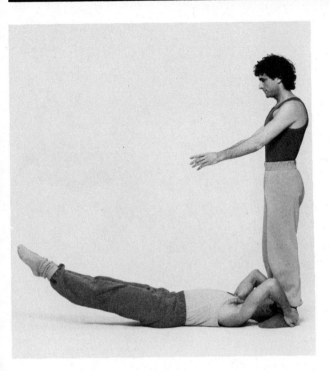

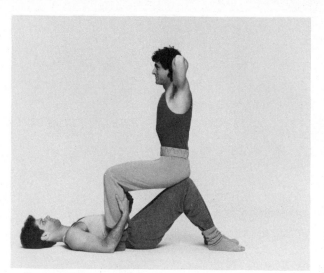 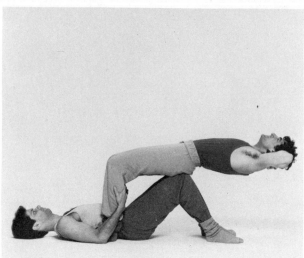

ADVANCED ABDOMEN

Roman Chair

The assisting partner lies on his back, knees bent, clasping your calves, as shown. Sit on his thighs, just below his knees, clasping your hands together behind your head, elbows open. Keeping a straight spine, bend back from the hips, until your body is parallel to the floor. Bend back up from the hips to return to starting position.

Breathing: Exhale as you go back, inhale as you rise.
Reps: 20 times; then exchange places with your partner.

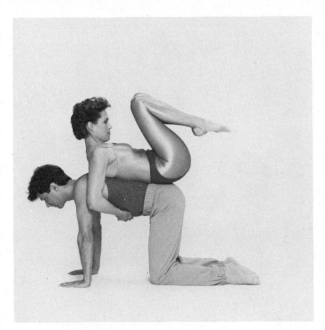 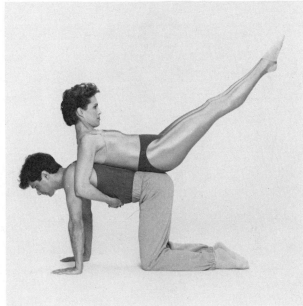

ADVANCED ABDOMEN

Reclining Double Leg Extension

The assisting partner kneels with his knees directly under his hips and his hands under his shoulders. Keep arms and back straight. Lie on the assisting partner's back, clasping your hands under his abdomen. Begin by bending the knees to the chest. Using your arms for support and balance, extend both legs to a 45° angle. Do not arch your back. Bend the knees back to the chest and repeat.

Breathing: Exhale as you extend, inhale as you bend.
Reps: 20 times; exchange places with your partner.

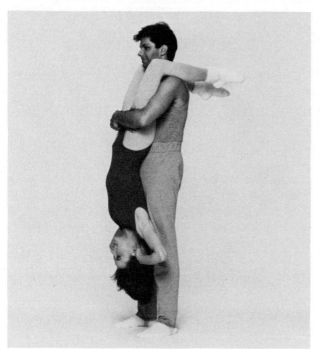 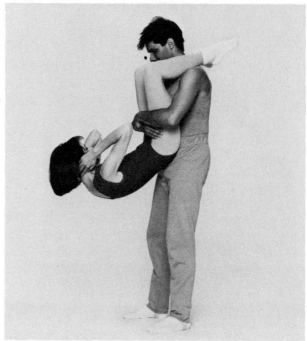

ADVANCED ABDOMEN

Standing Antigravitational Sit-up

Clasp your calves over your partner's neck and shoulders. Lace your fingers behind your head, elbows open. The assisting partner wraps his arms over your thighs for support. In a slow four-count motion, curl up your spine, bringing your elbows to your knees. Lower in four counts, then repeat.

Breathing: Exhale as you rise, inhale as you lower.
Reps: As many times as you can.

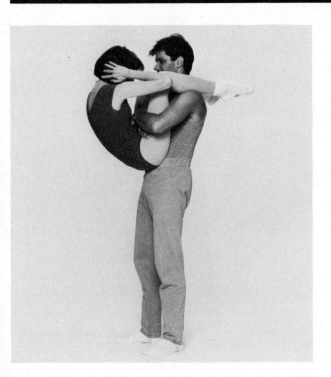

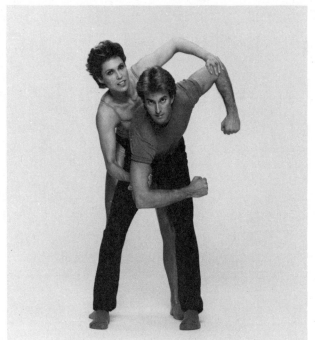 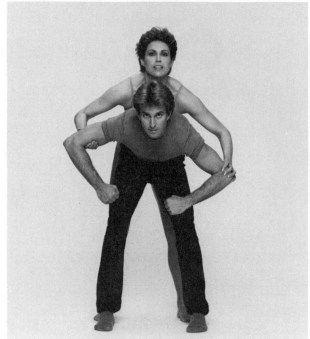

ABDOMEN

Oblique Side Twist
(works obliques)

This exercise is performed the same way as the first post-routine Negative Emphasis exercise (Chapter 7), except both partners are bent over from the hips and knees.

Breathing: Exhale on twist.
Reps: 20 times; then change positions with your partner.

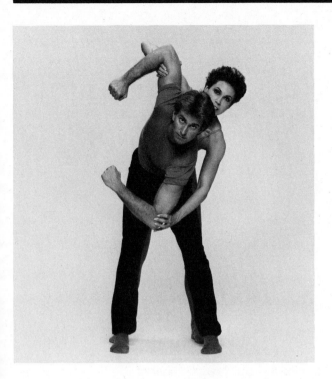

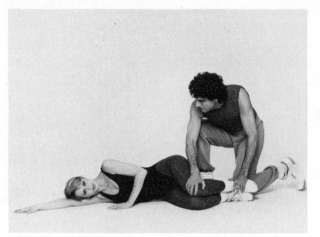 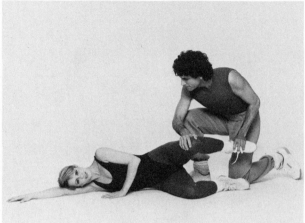

LEG

Lying, Bent-Knee Side Leg Lift
(works outer thigh and buttocks)

Lying on your side, bend your legs at right angles to your hips, as shown. The assisting partner kneels behind you, placing one hand on the working knee, the other on the foot. With resistance created from your partner, press your knee up as hard as you can. Resist on the way down as well. Do not lean back from the hips.

Breathing: Exhale as you lift, inhale as you lower.
Reps: 15 times per leg.

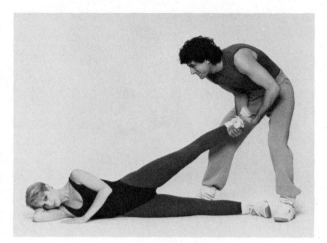 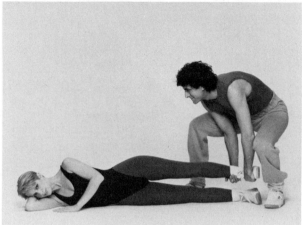

LEG

Lying Straight Leg Adduction
(works inner thigh)

Lie on your side with straight legs extended directly beneath. Begin with the working leg raised 2 feet. The assisting partner places both his hands under your ankle and creates resistance with his arms and body as you lower your leg. Release and return to starting position.

Breathing: Exhale as you lower, inhale as you rise.
Reps: 15 times per leg.

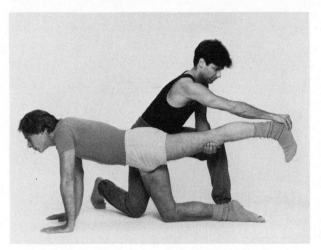 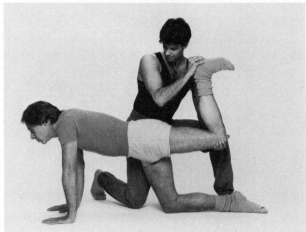

LEGS

Isolated Hamstring Curl
(works hamstrings)

Kneel on one knee, placing the hands directly under your shoulders. Lift the working leg parallel to the floor. The assisting partner kneels next to you, placing one hand under the working knee, and the other hand on your heel. Isolating the movement from the knee, bring the heel to a 90° position against your partner's hand resistance. Do not arch back! Lower Lower leg and repeat.

Breathing: Exhale on the way up, inhale on the way down.
Reps: 12 times, and change legs.

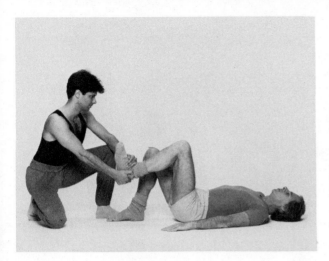 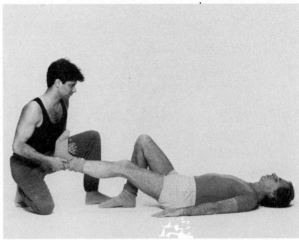

HIPS

Lying Hip Flexion
(works hip flexors)

Lie on your back, arms by your side, working leg extended. With resistance from your partner's hands, as shown, pull the knee toward the chest. Release and repeat.

Breathing: Exhale as the knee moves toward chest, inhale as the knee moves away from the chest.

Reps: 12 times per leg.

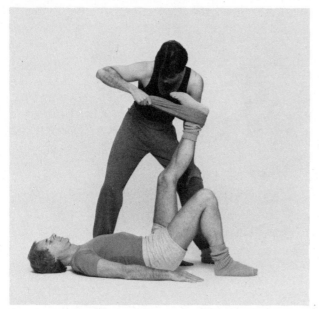 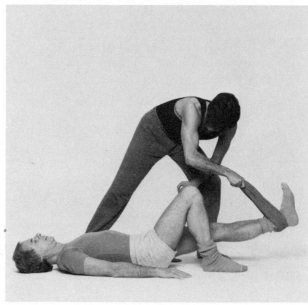

HIPS

Lying Hip Extension
(works hip extensors)

Lie on your back, arms by your side, working leg extended 90° to your body, as shown. The assisting partner wraps a towel around the back of your ankle and creates resistance with his arms and body weight as you bring your heel to the floor. Lift and repeat.

Breathing: Exhale as you lower, inhale as you rise.
Reps: 12 times and change legs.

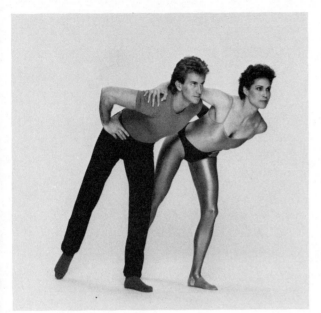 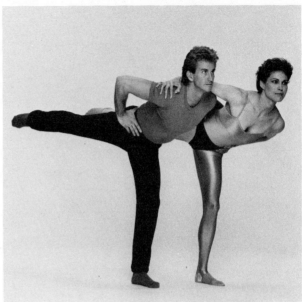

HIPS AND BACK

Bent-over Straight Leg Raise
(works hips and back)

Stand, side by side, bent over from the waist. Wrap your outside arm around your partner's torso and place the other hand on your hip. Bend the front knee and extend the other leg behind you, as shown. Simultaneously lift the back leg until parallel to the floor. Lower and repeat.

Breathing: Exhale as you lift up, inhale as you lower.
Reps: 15 times per leg.

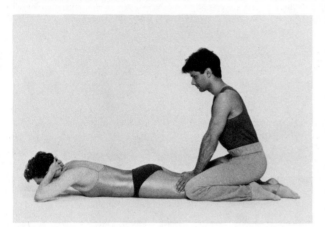 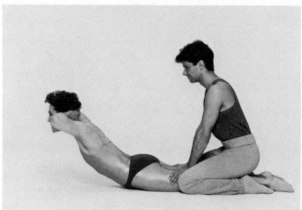

BACK

Lying Hyperextensions
(upper and lower back)

Lie on the floor, face down, legs together. Lace your fingers behind the back of your head, as shown. The assisting partner straddles your legs, placing his hands on the back of your thighs. Lift your torso off the floor as high as you can. Lower and repeat.

Breathing: Exhale as you lift, inhale as you lower.
Reps: 12 times.

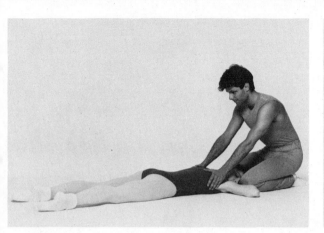 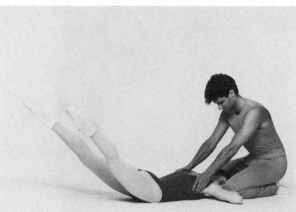

BACK

Lower Back Hyperextension
(works lower back)

This exercise is to be performed the same way as the previous hyperextension, except you lift your legs instead of your torso. The assisting partner places his hands on your shoulder blades. You place your hands on the floor under your head.

Breathing: Exhale as you lift, inhale as you lower.
Reps: 12 times.

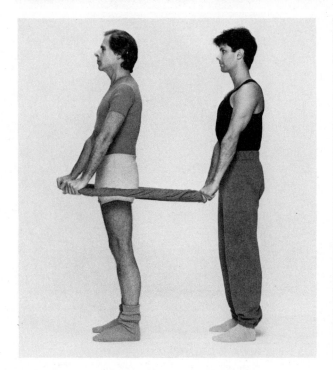 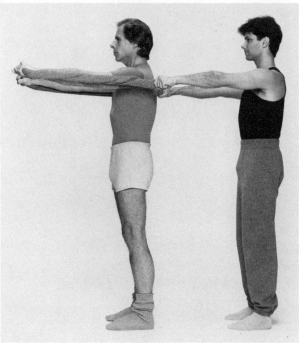

SHOULDERS

Standing Front Lateral Raise
(works anterior deltoids)

Stand facing the same direction, about 3 feet apart. Each partner, holding the ends of 2 towels, slowly raises the arms in front until reaching shoulder height, parallel to the floor. Resistance is created by the partner standing behind on the way up and by the partner in front on the way down. Do not lean with the body.

Breathing: Exhale on the way up, inhale on the way down.
Reps: 12 times; then exchange places with your partner.

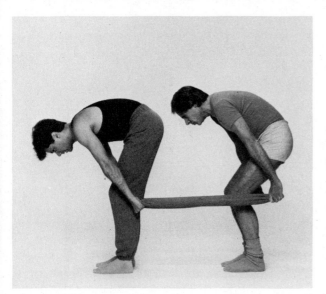 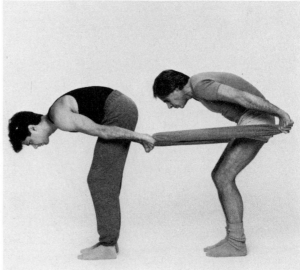

SHOULDERS

Bent-over Rear Lateral Raise
(works posterior deltoid)

This exercise is done the same way as the preceding anterior deltoid
exercise, with the exception that both partners are bent over from the hip
and the movement extends to the rear, parallel to the floor. The same
resistance is created, back and forth. Do not lean forward.

Breathing: Exhale on the way back, inhale on the way forward.
Reps: 12 times; exchange places with your partner.

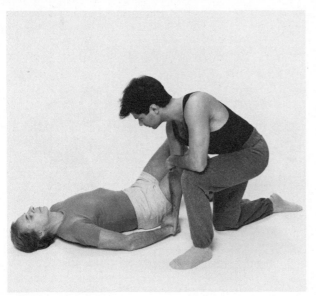
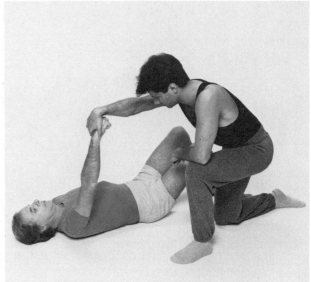

SHOULDER

One Arm Front Lateral Raise
(works anterior deltoid)

Lie on your back, knees bent, working arm on floor next to your side. The assisting partner, kneeling next to you, clasps his hand over your fist and creates smooth resistance as you lift your arm to a perpendicular position. Release to floor and repeat.

Breathing: Exhale on the way up, inhale on the way down.
Reps: 12 times; then change arms.

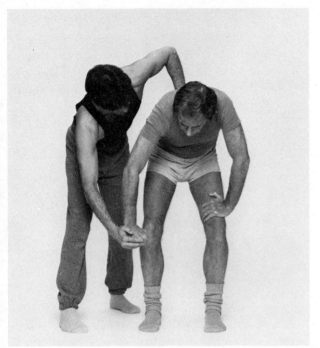 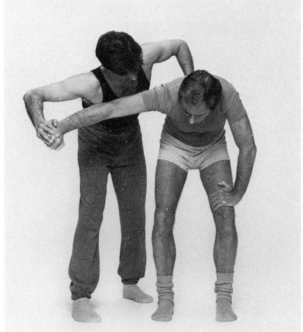

SHOULDER AND MIDDLE BACK

Bent-over One Arm Side Lateral Raise
(works rhomboids)

Bend over from the hips and extend the working arm directly under shoulder, as shown. Keep elbow slightly bent. The assisting partner stands next to you, clasps your fist, and creates resistance as you slowly extend your arm to a position parallel to the floor.

Breathing: Exhale on the way up, inhale on the way down.
Reps: 12 times.

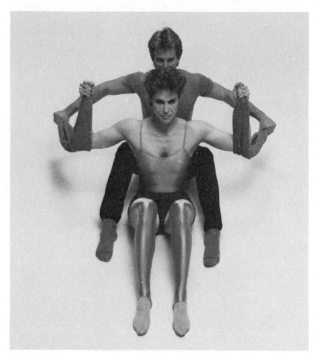
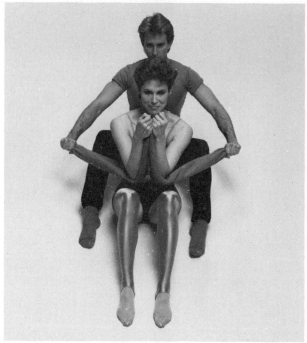

CHEST

Double "Pec-Dec"
(works pectorals)

Sit facing the same direction, knees bent. Holding 2 towels wrapped over your forearms, lift the arms, elbows bent, parallel to the floor, as shown. The assisting partner, holding the other ends of the towels, creates resistance as you bring your parallel forearms together until they touch. The assisting partner then pulls your arms back open as you resist until you return to starting position. Keep strict form. Do not lower the elbows.

Breathing: Exhale as the arms are brought together, inhale as they open.
Reps: 12 times.

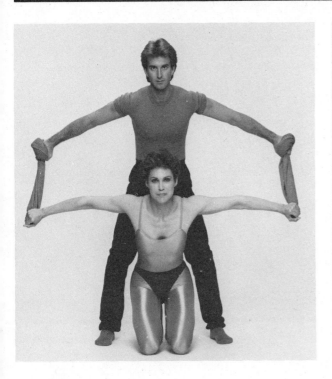 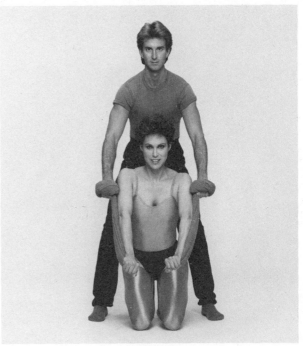

CHEST

Double Cable Fly
(works pectorals)

Begin in a kneeling position, clasping the ends of 2 towels, arms open, as shown. The assisting partner stands behind and, clasping the other ends of the towels, creates resistance as you bring your hands together. He then pulls back to starting position, as you resist. Keep your elbows slightly bent and isolate the movement from the shoulder joint.

Breathing: Exhale as the arms are brought together, inhale as they open.
Reps: 12 times.

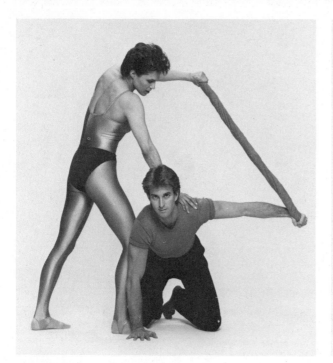
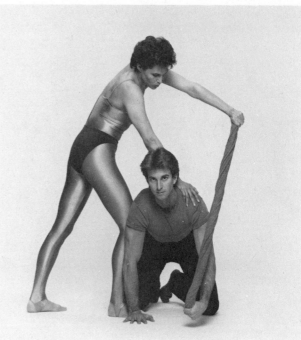

CHEST

Single Cable Fly
(works pectorals)

This exercise is performed the same way as the Double Cable Fly, except with one arm at a time. The assisting partner stands to the side, placing her other hand on the back of your shoulder for support and balance.

Breathing: Exhale as the arm is brought down, inhale as the arm is brought up.
Reps: 12 times for each arm.

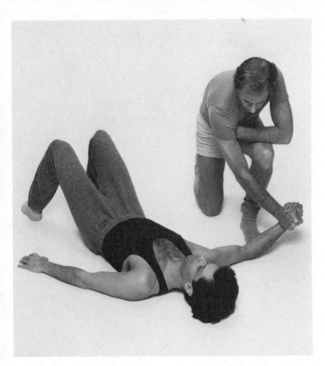
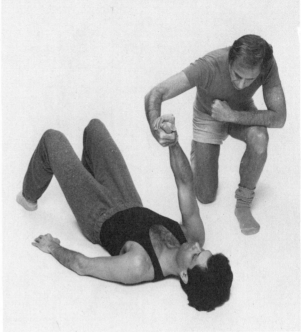

CHEST

One Arm Fly
(works pectorals)

This exercise is performed the same way as the Single Cable Fly, except you lie on your back, knees bent, and your partner kneels facing you. Begin with the working arm open and cross over your chest. Resistance is created in both directions.

Breathing: Exhale on the way up, inhale as you lower.
Reps: 12 times and change arms.

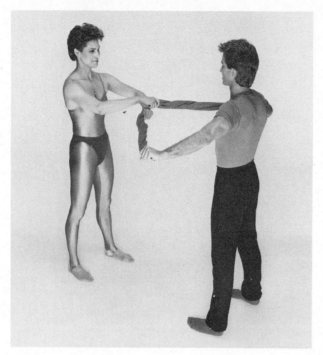 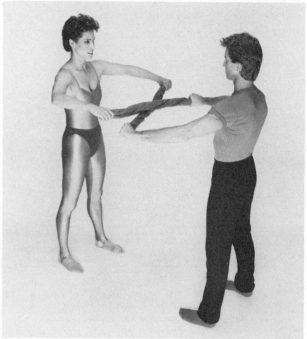

CHEST

Standing Double Cross Cable Fly
(works chest and back)

This exercise is performed the same way as the standing/lying Cross Cable Pull (Chapter 7). However, resistance is created in both directions with this exercise. Do not lean forward or backward. Isolate movement from shoulders.

Breathing: Exhale as you close the arms, inhale as they open.
Reps: 12 times, crossing the arms.

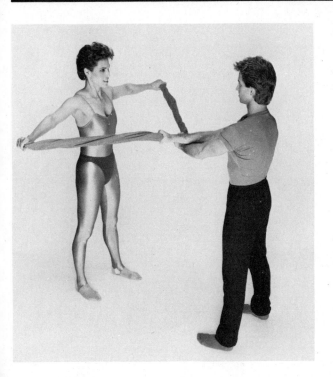

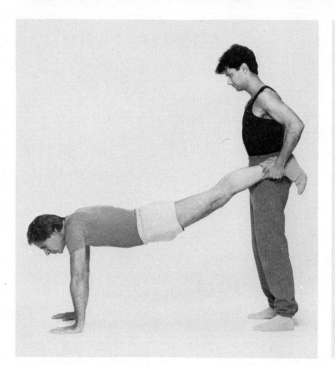
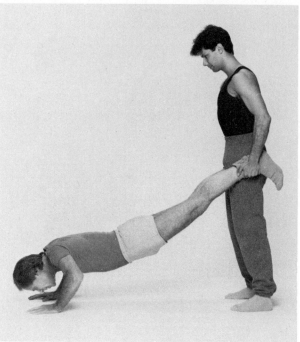

CHEST

Incline Push-up
(works upper pectorals)

Position your arms into a push-up placement. (See the freebody exercises in Chapter 3 for isolating specific upper body and arm muscles.) The assisting partner, standing behind you, picks up your legs by the ankles, as shown. Lower your arms and lower your head and chest to the floor. Push back up and repeat.

Breathing: Exhale on the way down, inhale on the way up.
Reps: As many times as you can.

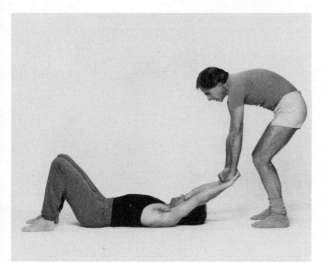 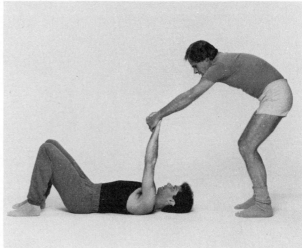

CHEST

Double Arm Pull-over
(works pectorals and latissimus dorsi)

Lie on your back, knees bent, arms extended back overhead. The assisting partner stands facing you, bending from the knees and hips. Clasping your hands, he creates resistance as you pull your stiff arms, isolated from the shoulder, and perpendicular, as shown. Your partner then pulls your arms back down to the starting position, as you resist.

Breathing: Exhale as you pull up, inhale as you lower.
Reps: 12 times.

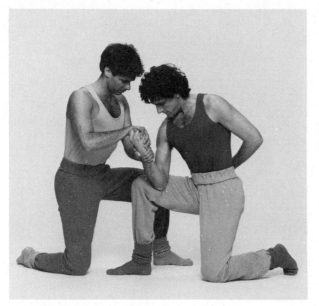 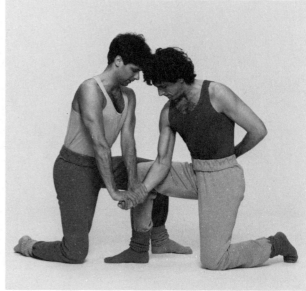

ARMS

Concentration Curl
(works bicep)

Kneel at right angles to your partner. Place your elbow inside your thigh, as shown. The assisting partner, clasping both hands over your wrist and fist, presses down until your arm is fully extended. With resistance, curl forearm back up to a flexed position and repeat.

Breathing: Exhale as the bicep is extended, inhale as the bicep is flexed.
Reps: 12 times per arm.

Note: Assisting partner gets negative tricep work.

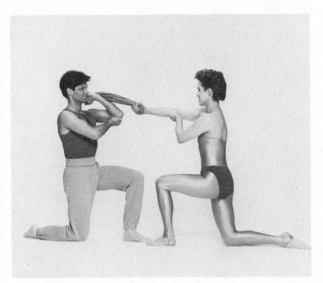 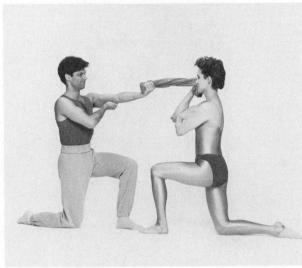

ARMS

Kneeling Bicep Cable Pull
(works bicep)

Kneel on one knee, facing your partner, as shown. Extend your right arm out in front of your body, parallel to the floor. Place your left hand on your right elbow to help isolate the bicep. Clasping a towel, begin with one partner flexing and one partner extending the arm. Alternate back and forth arm movements.

Breathing: Exhale as you extend, inhale as you bend your arm.
Reps: 12 times and change arms.

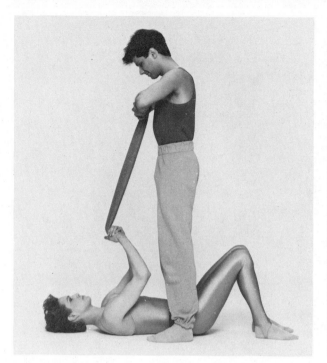 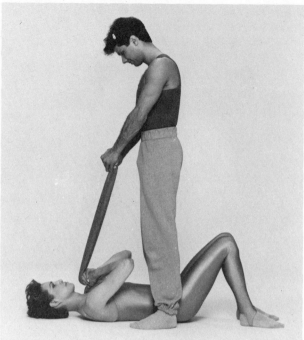

ARM AND SHOULDERS

Mixed Arm and Shoulder
(works trapezius and biceps)

Lie on your back, knees bent, arms extended at a 45° angle, clasping the
end of a towel. Your partner stands over you, straddling your hips, holding
the other end of the towel in an upright row position (see the Double
Upright Row in Chapter 4). As you bend your arms (working your bicep),
your partner extends his arms (working his shoulder). In isolated
movements, alternate up and down, curls and rows.

Breathing: Exhale as you flex, inhale as you extend.
Reps: 12 times.

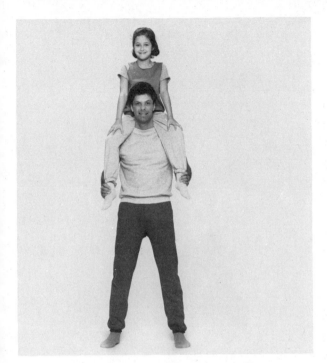 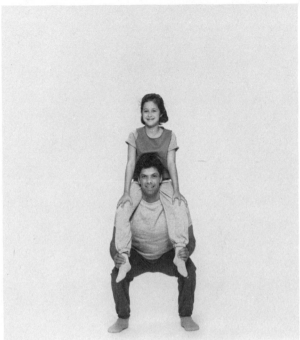

SPECIAL PARTNERS

Working out with "little partners" can be fun, too. Incorporate the children in your life into your fitness routines. Working out together provides an additional activity to share. Children love to touch. Exercise for children builds confidence, body awareness, and self-esteem.

Squats
(works adult's thighs/child's balance)

Stand with legs open, feet pointed to the front. The assisting "little partner" sits on your shoulders. Bend your knees until your thighs are parallel to the floor. Stand back up and repeat.

Breathing: Exhale as you lower, inhale as you stand up.
Reps: 20 times.

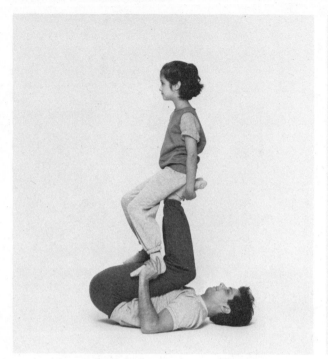 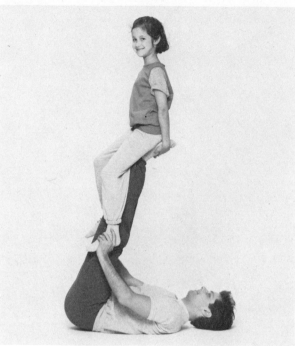

Leg Presses
(works adult's thighs/child's balance)

Lie on your back, knees on your chest. The assisting "little partner" sits squarely on your feet. Clasp each other's feet for support and balance. Extend the leg straight up, pushing your "little partner's" body weight.

Breathing: Inhale as you lower, exhale as you press.
Reps: 20 times.

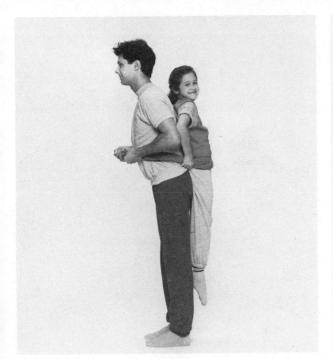
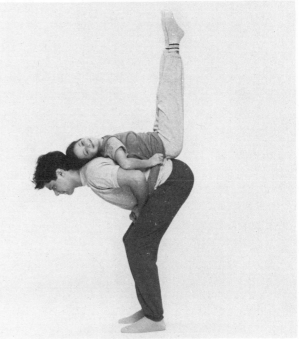

Bent-over Leg Raise

(works adult's back and legs/child's stomach and legs)

Stand facing opposite directions. Wrap a towel around your "little partner's" hips and lift her off the floor. Holding her securely with the towel, bend your knees and hips until your back is parallel to the floor. At the same time, she extends her legs straight up. Straighten your back and knees and repeat.

Breathing: Exhale as you go over, inhale on the way up.
Reps: 12 times.

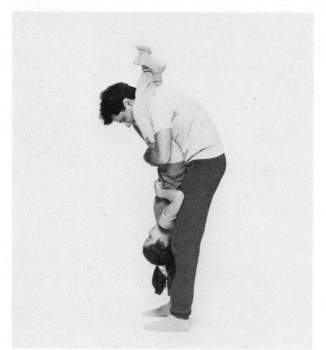 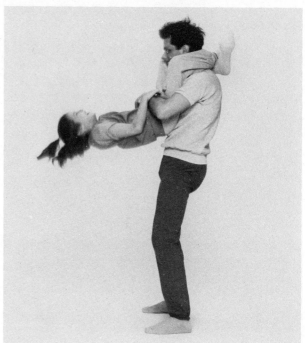

Stomach Swing
(works adult's back/child's abdomen)

Stand, legs open 1 foot. Pick your "little partner" up, upside down, so she can wrap her feet around your neck and shoulders, as shown. Wrap your arm around her hips. In a swinging motion, lift your "little partner" up and down.

Breathing: Rhythmically.
Reps: 20 times.

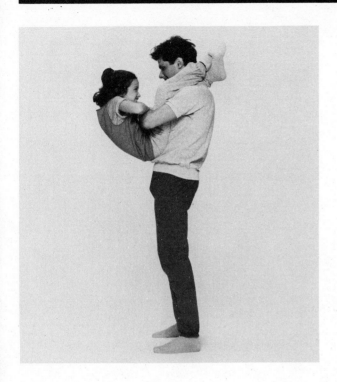

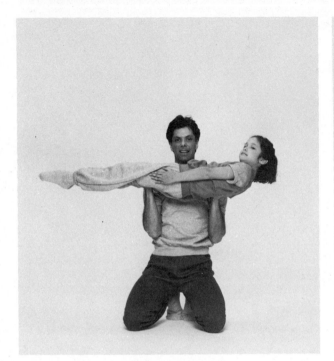 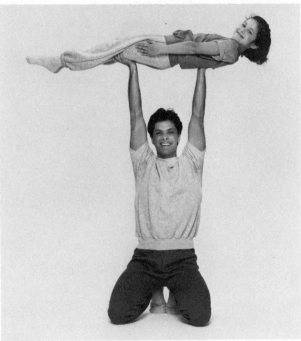

Military Press
(works adult's shoulders/child's abdomen)

Kneel, holding your "little partner's" body under her legs and middle back. Press her straight up overhead.

Breathing: Exhale as you rise, inhale as you lower.
Reps: 20 times.

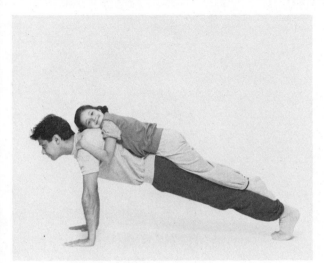 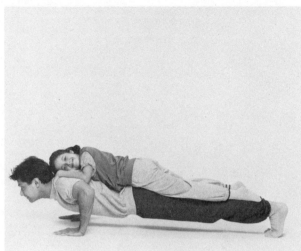

Assisted Push-up
(works adult's arms and shoulders)

Place hands on floor outside shoulders. Keeping your feet together and body straight, press up and down. Have your "little partner" lie on your back for additional resistance.

Breathing: Inhale as you lower, exhale as you push up.
Reps: 20 times.

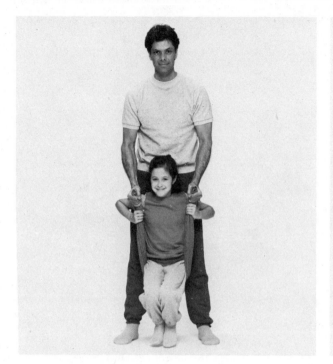 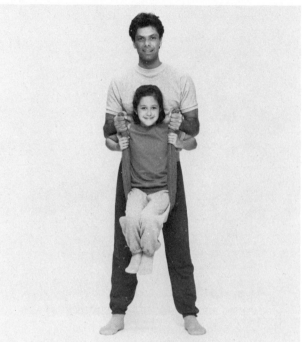

Bicep Curl
(works adult's arms)

Stand holding the ends of a towel. The assisting "little partner" sits in the middle of the towel, as shown. Starting with your arms extended, bend your elbows and lift your seated "little partner." Lower your arms and repeat.

Breathing: Exhale as you lower, inhale as you rise.
Reps: 12 times.

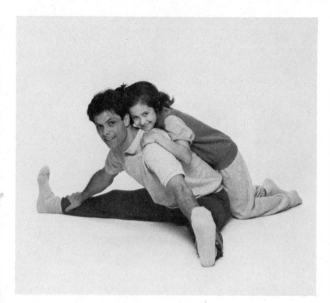 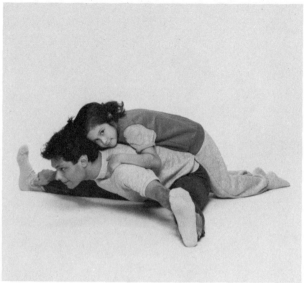

Straddle Stretch
(works adult's inner thighs)

Sit on the floor, legs straddled, clasping your ankles. The assisting "little partner" lies on your back, as shown. As you lean forward to stretch, your "little partner" leans with you, providing a little extra resistance.

Breathing: Exhale as you bend forward, inhale as you go up.
Reps: 6 times.

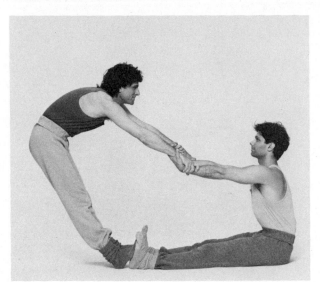 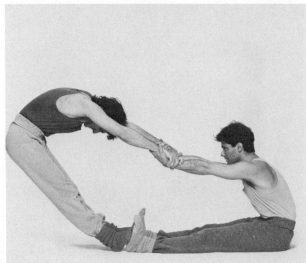

FLEXIBILITY EXERCISES

The following 5 stretching exercises can be added to or substituted within the Basic, Aerobic and Advanced Programs. They are a little more advanced, so be sure to work up to them slowly.

Leaning "Lat" Pull

(works hamstrings, calves, upper back, and arms)

The assisting partner sits on the floor first, extending straight parallel legs. Begin by bracing your feet against your partner's, as shown. Clasp your partner's wrist, lean back, and slowly lower the hips. Drop the head. Pull back up and repeat.

Breathing: Exhale on the way down, inhale on the way up.
Reps: 6 times, holding for 10 seconds.

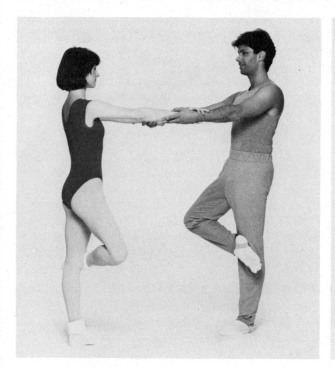 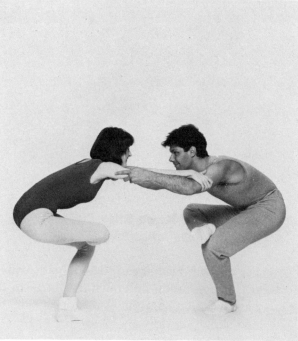

Standing Half-Lotus
(works buttocks)

Stand facing the same direction, 3 to 4 feet apart, clasping your partner's
arms. Bending one knee, fold it across your standing leg, as shown. Using
each other's arms for balance and support, bend the standing leg into a
squatting position. Stand back up and repeat.

Breathing: Exhale as you lower, inhale as you come up.
Reps: 6 times per leg.

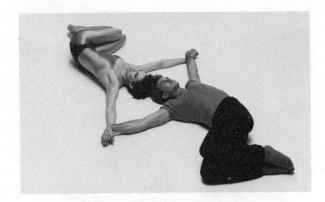 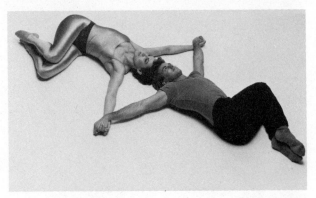

Lying Bent-Knee Side Twist
(works hip and abdomen)

Lie on your back, head to head with your partner. Extend the arms to the side, clasp hands, and bend the knees to the chest. Simultaneously alternate twisting from the hips, side to side. Stretch slowly, keeping the arms and shoulders down.

Breathing: Exhale in rhythm with the twist.
Reps: Twist to each side 6 times.

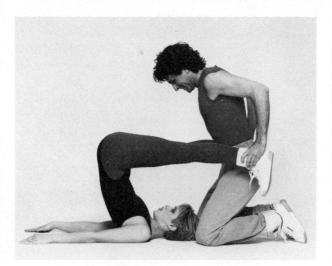
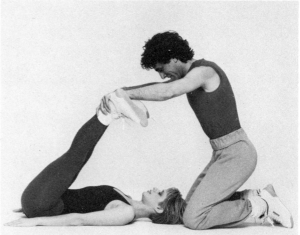

Straddle Plough
(works back and hamstrings)

Lie on your back, straddle your legs open and roll up onto your shoulders. The assisting partner kneels behind you and places his hands on your ankles. Keeping your legs open and as straight as possible, slowly roll down your spinal column while your partner places *gentle* resistance on your legs. Roll back to the shoulders and repeat.

Breathing: Exhale on the way down, inhale on the way up.
Reps: 6 times.

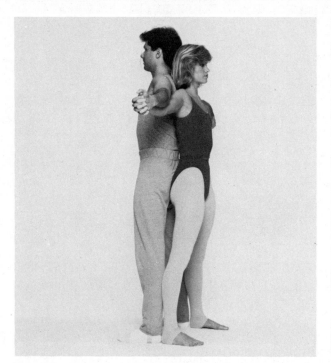
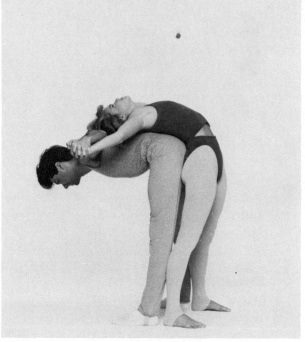

Standing Back-Arch
(works abdomen and lower back)

This exercise is done the same way as the Sitting Abdominal/Inner Thigh Stretch (see Pre-routine Stretch #2 in Chapter 4), except that both partners are standing.

Breathing: Exhale on the stretch, inhale on the release.
Reps: 6 times; then exchange places with your partner.

9 Training and Overtraining

Working out can change your life. The realization that you have the ability to alter your physical appearance and level of energy can have an astounding psychological effect. It gives you a sense of control over your life. You begin to change bad habits. You create a healthy lifestyle. You become addicted to feeling good, to experiencing the effects of training.

Physiologists have coined the term *training effect* to define the body's adaptation to any methodical application of overload—overload being any specific form of *stress* that we want the body to respond to.

Stress is an interesting phenomenon. According to Dr. Hans Selye, a noted authority on stress, there are basically two categories: distress and eustress. Distress occurs when we are upset, that is, angry, fearful, or tense. Eustress occurs when we are elated, that is, joyful or excited, even when we are being creative. Both emotional states create bodily tension. Similar biochemical reactions occur within the body, that is, increased adrenalin flow, dilated blood vessels, increased heart rate, elevated blood sugar, dilated pupils, and slowed digestion.

Work done during exercise creates the same stimulus and produces the same chemical reactions as distress and eustress. In other words, the body's chemical regulators do not differentiate the source of stress. If we did not have a discerning intelligence, our body would not know the difference between being in the woods running away from a bear and being in our living room running on a treadmill. It goes without saying, however, that we would feel different emotionally in each of these situations, which would undoubtedly affect our performance.

In any case, with our higher intelligence, we can control our undiscriminating chemical plants and muscle reactions. We have an almost unlimited ability to adjust to different forms of work overload if we train appropriately. We can selectively and systematically increase our strength, stamina, agility, and mental alertness. Last year, a young circus performer completed a quadruple somersault during a trapeze act. This feat had long been considered impossible. Human motivation creates limitless possibilities. Herein lies the potential danger. We are human. Our addiction to feeling good and gaining control over our lives through physical training can lead to overtraining. More is *not* necessarily better.

Overtraining can lead to physical and mental exhaustion. Exhaustion is the body's built-in defense mechanism to say it's had enough. Stress is the stimulus, adaptation is the training effect, overtraining is exhaustion. You may begin to lose your appetite, become easily tired, and require more sleep and enjoy working out less. More severe warning signs include headaches, weight loss, increased or decreased blood pressure or resting pulse rate, swollen lymph nodes, and constipation or diarrhea. Your digestive system shuts down. Accumulation of metabolic waste products such as lactic, pyruvic, and succinic acids, which lower muscle pH (ratio of alkalinity to acidity), begins to inhibit metabolism, causing severe soreness and stiffness. Depletion of carbohydrate sources (muscle and liver glycogen and glucose) prevents further energy resynthesis. Hormonal imbalances also occur. The adrenals can actually go into total remission if high-intensity workouts are continued for too long.

To avoid overtraining, you must balance your workouts with rest and recuperation for mind and body. Include active and passive relaxation techniques. Active rest might include hiking, leisure cycling, or similar outdoor activities where fresh air can be breathed, and sunshine—in moderate doses—can be absorbed, which can stimulate hormone production. Passive relaxation might include treating yourself to a massage or soaking in a hot tub with mineral salts.

Balance in training is the key.

Appendix: Muscle Identification

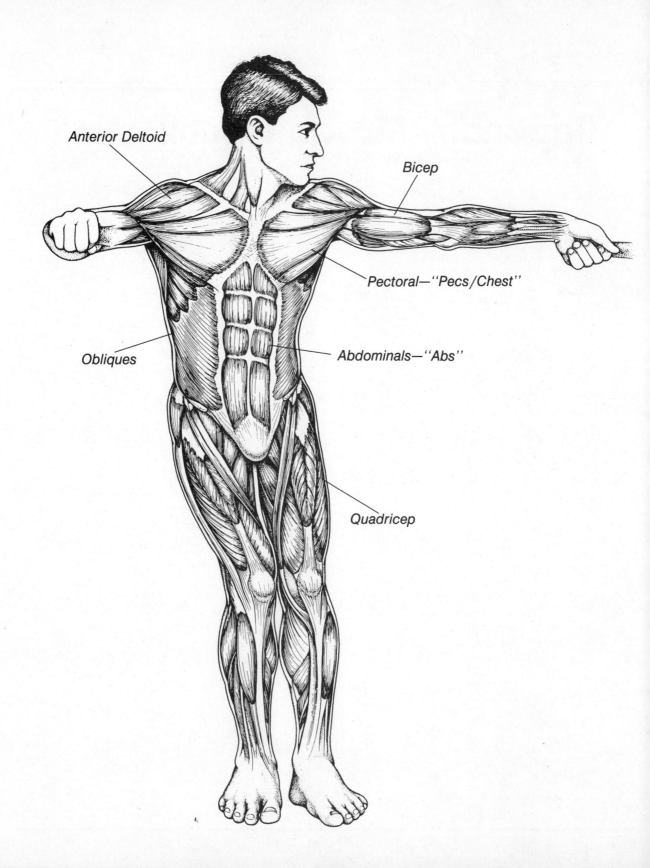

Anterior Deltoid

Bicep

Pectoral—"Pecs/Chest"

Obliques

Abdominals—"Abs"

Quadricep

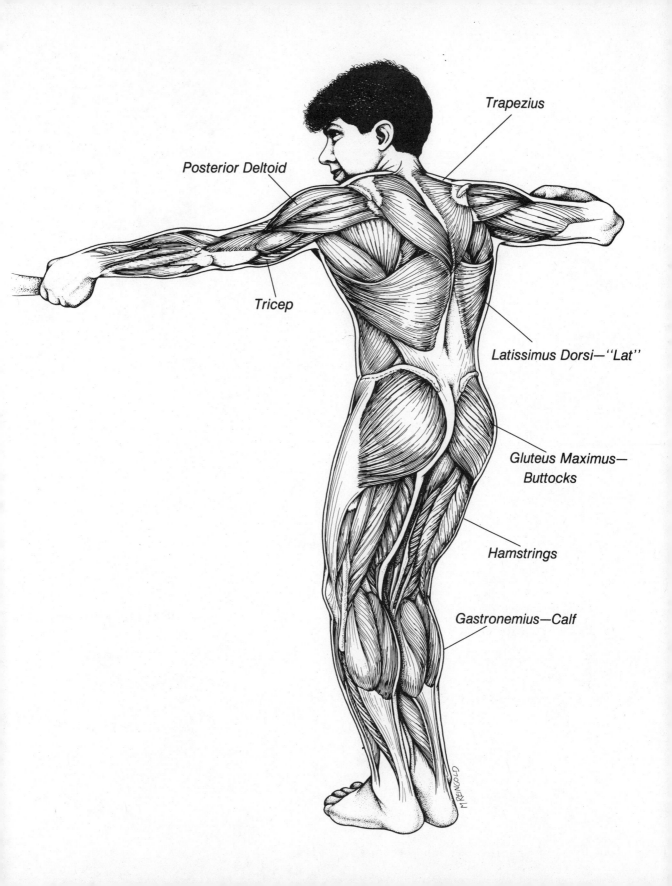

Trapezius

Posterior Deltoid

Tricep

Latissimus Dorsi—"Lat"

Gluteus Maximus—
Buttocks

Hamstrings

Gastronemius—Calf

M.REINGOLD